The New Mobile Age

HOW TECHNOLOGY WILL EXTEND THE HEALTHSPAN AND OPTIMIZE THE LIFESPAN

Joseph C. Kvedar MD

Carol Colman and Gina Cella
Partners Connected Health

Partners Connected Health
25 New Chardon Street, 3rd Floor, Suite 300
Boston, MA 02114
Printed in the United States of America
Partners Connected Health
First Printing, 2017
ISBN: 0692906843
ISBN 13: 9780692906842

The New Mobile Age

**HOW TECHNOLOGY WILL EXTEND THE HEALTHSPAN
AND OPTIMIZE THE LIFESPAN**

Contents

Acknowledgments

This book represents a true collaboration. The contributions of my co-authors, Carol Colman and Gina Cella, can't be overstated. With all going on in our collective busy lives, writing this book became a true passion—and a continuation of our journey to advance the application of innovative connected health solutions to solve critical challenges in healthcare delivery. This book is a tribute to the strength of the team.

I am thrilled that my friend and colleague Charlotte Yeh agreed to write the Foreword. Her dedication to longevity has been impressive and the book would be far less impactful without her involvement.

I must acknowledge the support of my family. My wife, Vicki, not only puts up with my overcommitted professional life, but enthusiastically supports me; likewise, with my incredibly successful adult children, Derek, Julie and Megan. Professional growth is easier to accomplish in the context of a loving, supportive family and I am blessed with one.

Why have I spent the last 33 years of my career at one institution? Chiefly because the environment at Partners HealthCare is one that prizes innovation and novel thinking. From inspirational mentors and teachers to insightful business leaders and world-class healthcare providers, I have been given the opportunity to help build a new model for care delivery.

My thanks to Drs. Gregg Meyer and David Torchiana for supporting me and encouraging me to contribute to connected health thought leadership on behalf of Partners HealthCare. No professional experience can compare to working for Gregg and Torch. Most of us in academia have more than one supervisor and the chair of my clinical department (Massachusetts General Hospital Department of Dermatology), Dr. David Fisher, has been enormously supportive over the years, despite the fact that my area of interest is not directly in dermatology.

I'm blessed to be surrounded by incredible talent at Partners Connected Health. All of our 60+ team members contributed in some way to this book. Their careful innovative work in design, clinical research, data science and implementation is bringing the vision of time-and-place-independent care to life. All of the sections of this book on chronic illness management and wellness are heavily influenced by what I've learned from working with this team.

I'm grateful to the community of thought leaders in aging for welcoming me to their banquet. When we started thinking about this book, we knew that we had many novel ideas to contribute to this important area, but we came at it from the experience and insights we have accumulated in connected health. We believe there are significant opportunities to apply connected health strategies to help our aging population live healthier longer, and this is acknowledged by the important advances and novel programs described in this book. Not only did aging experts, healthcare innovators and others redefining how we manage our golden years willingly interview for the book, but they've warmly welcomed us into the community.

I've compared our style of assembling the content for this book to that of an investigative reporter. As every writer knows, a good copy editor is invaluable and I'd like to thank ours, Marya Dalrymple. And without the contributions of those individuals we interviewed, there would be no book. Their varied opinions and experiences are what makes for an interesting and dynamic read. To that end, I wish to thank everyone listed here for their insights and thoughtful contributions: Michael Birt, PhD, principal, Blue Triangle; Christine Cassel, MD, planning dean, Kaiser Permanente Medical School; Eric Dishman, director, *All of Us*, NIH; Sean Duffy, co-founder and CEO, Omada Health; Rana el Kaliouby, PhD, CEO, Affectiva; Rushika Fernandopulle, MD, MPP, co-founder and CEO, Iora Health; Ted Fischer, vice president, Business Development, Hasbro, Inc.; Michael Greeley, co-founder, Flare Capital Partners; Jim Harper, PhD, co-founder, Sonde Health; Rob Havasy, MS, senior director, HIS, HIMSS North America; Jody Holtzman, senior vice president, Market Innovation, AARP; Kamal Jethwani, MD, MPH, senior director, Connected Health Innovation, Partners HealthCare; Lindsay Jurist-Rosner, co-founder and CEO, Wellthy; Cory Kidd, PhD, founder and CEO, Catalia Health; Eric S. Kim, PhD, Center for Health and Happiness, Harvard School of Public Health; Daniel Kraft, MD, chair for medicine, Singularity University; Dennis Lally, co-founder, Rendever; Laura Landro, journalist; Bruce Leff, MD, director, The Center for Transformative Geriatric Research and professor of medicine, Johns Hopkins Medicine; Calum MacRae, MD, PhD, chief of Cardiovascular Medicine, Brigham and Women's Hospital and head of the One Brave Idea research project; Tom Nesbitt, MD, MPH, associate vice Chancellor for Strategic Technologies and Alliances, UC Davis Health; Adam Pellegrini, general manager, Fitbit Health Solutions; Reena Sanger, head, Digital and Connected Health, Ipsos Healthcare; Lisa Suennen, senior managing director, Healthcare, GE Ventures and managing partner, Venture Valkyrie; S. Shyam Sundar, PhD, distinguished professor and founding director, Media Effects Research Lab, Penn State University's College of Communications;

Rudolph E. Tanzi, PhD, vice-chair, Neurology Department, and director, Genetics and Aging Research Unit, Massachusetts General Hospital;

Sarah Thomas, senior director of Global Innovation, Genesis Rehab Services/Genesis Healthcare, and executive-in residence and innovation fellow, Aging2.0; Bradley Merrill Thompson, digital health and combination product regulatory attorney, Epstein Becker & Green, P.C.; Thuc Vu, PhD, co-founder, Ohmnilabs; Victor Wang, CEO, care. coach; Heather M. Young, PhD, RN, FAAN, founding dean, Betty Irene Moore School of Nursing, UC Davis Health System.

The following individuals also gave of their time and offered wisdom that helped shape the book's content: E. Ray Dorsey, MD, professor of Neurology and director, Center for Human Experimental Therapeutics (CHET), University of Rochester Medical Center; Tony Fantana, PhD; Craig Fontenot, former vice president, Product Strategy & Development, AARP; Ryan R. Fortna, MD, PhD, pathologist, Northwest Pathology; Adam Gazzaley, MD, PhD, professor, Neurology, Physiology and Psychiatry, UCSF, founder/executive director, Neuroscape, and co-founder and chief science advisor, Akili Interactive Labs; Denise M. Kalos, COO, Affirmativ Health; Sarah Lenz Lock, JD, senior vice president for Policy, AARP's Policy, Research and International Affairs, and executive director, Global Council on Brain Health; Scott Newland, senior UX/UI designer, Partners Connected Health.

We will all continue to hear more, learn more and create more innovative solutions that support healthy aging and, in the process, improve healthcare for all ages. I hope this book inspires greater understanding and focus when it comes to creating the right tools for healthy longevity.

FOREWORD

What is Old?

By Charlotte S. Yeh, MD, Chief Medical Officer, AARP Services, Inc.

I turned 65 this year, a milestone birthday in that I—a former staff physician and chief of the Department of Emergency Medicine at two major Boston hospitals, who now serves as chief medical officer for AARP Services, Inc.—had to face the fact that it was time for me to enroll in Medicare. As a former Boston Regional Administrator for the Centers for Medicare and Medicaid Services, I had helped many a friend and family member through the Medicare enrollment process. Now, much to my surprise, it was my turn: But this time, it was different—it was *personal*.

Like many of us, I looked in the mirror and said to myself, "Am I really that old?" Because I certainly don't feel old. I'm still vibrant, living life to the fullest, working hard and enjoying friends and family. How could I possibly have reached that landmark number that is synonymous with "old?"

Many ask this same question. After all, every two days 20,000 people in the United States will join me when they turn 65. We all have a lot to look forward to since the fastest growing segment of our population is people 85 and older, followed by the second fastest growing segment—people who are 100 and older. If so many of us are living longer, isn't it time we reconsider what it means to be old? Maybe, we are defining age too narrowly. . . . Age really is just a number—but a number that reflects experience, knowledge, a life's journey with twists and turns, successes, failures and lessons learned. Rather than express dismay at reaching the age of 65, shouldn't we be embracing our age?

In fact, long before I celebrated this momentous moment of 65, I had been exploring what is aging, what is old, what is meaningful to longevity, as part of my work with AARP Services, Inc., a subsidiary of AARP that oversees and manages the relationships with companies that provide AARP member benefits.

After reviewing the research literature, listening to the stories of AARP members and studying the engagement of people enrolled in Medicare, I have come to understand how exciting and contributory aging actually is.

While we think of innovation and entrepreneurialism as pertaining to the realm of the young, people in their 50s and 60s start businesses at nearly twice the rate of people in their 20s. When we look at the economy, individuals over 50 generate $7.6 trillion in annual economic activity, and are responsible for more than half of every dollar spent in the United States. Rather than an economic burden, this older generation is a significant contributor to the economy.

And when we look at ourselves, we find that our happiness increases, and moves steadily upward, surpassing the happiness of our youth. Moreover, neuroscience has shown that as one ages, one's brain demonstrates improved vocabulary, problem solving, pattern recognition, emotional stability and overall better executive function. In short, we do get wiser as we age.

The Importance of Resiliency

In the course of my every day work to "transform healthcare" at AARP Services, Inc., I have been translating research and data from health and well-being of the person into the business of healthcare. For instance, good health is not the end-goal for the consumer. Rather, living well on one's own terms is the end-goal, with the consumer looking at health as simply a tool to achieve a satisfied life.

Modern medicine has brought us extended longevity. Attention to social determinants such as food, security, jobs, education, transportation and livable communities have contributed to better health outcomes. But the real nugget behind aging wonderfully is resiliency—the ability and attitude that ensures you can cope and adapt when life slams you with a curve ball. What it takes to weather the times when "life happens" and recover when the winds of change blow and knock you down.

Reviewing the literature reveals that three components, in particular, inform the essence of resiliency: a strong sense of purpose, optimism about aging and social connections. A strong sense of purpose is associated with fewer heart attacks, strokes and cases of dementia, fewer nights in the hospital and lower healthcare costs. A positive view of aging has been correlated with a 44% increased likelihood of recovering fully from a severe disability, as well as fewer plaques and tangles in the brain, anatomic evidence associated with dementia. Loneliness, or the feeling of not being connected to others, has been shown to have a health risk equivalent to smoking 15 cigarettes a day. With these insights, is it any wonder that we should be pursuing resiliency as part of healthy longevity?

My appreciation for resiliency isn't only informed by my nearly 30 years of emergency medicine practice, decades of administrative health experience and the data and science. Six years ago, while crossing the street in a crosswalk with a green "walk" sign, a car plowed into me on a rainy evening in Washington, DC. I saw firsthand what happens when the unthinkable occurs in a split second, immediately changing how one lives; when you transition instantaneously and irrevocably from a "person" to a "patient." It was a real eye-opener.

I had always focused a great deal on patient empowerment and giving individuals a voice in their healthcare. This commitment is now also informed by my accident—I know what it's like to be frightened, in pain, utterly powerless and dependent. After the accident, I first faced the specter of being unable to care for myself, a life limited in activities and facing a new and different version of me: no longer a contributor, but a burden.

However, during the extended recovery process, these initial negative perceptions eroded away and disappeared. During this time, I learned the importance of attitude, adaptation and how to retain a sense of self that allows one to face personal change. My accident taught me what it means to navigate through the complexities of the fragmented health system, how hard it can be to communicate with doctors and what it means to be told what you can't do, instead of what you can do. The importance of resilience was revealed to me: Yes, there is my "new normal," accepting I will never be what I once was. . . . But resilience also meant never losing optimism: While I will never again be "normal," I can certainly aspire to "how close to normal can I get."

My experience caused me to shed long-held biases and assumptions and created opportunity for me to be open to new learnings. Despite years of training and experience as an emergency medicine physician, I learned things in my recovery that I never learned in medical school—about biomechanics, muscle group interaction and posture. Now I'm in better shape, I have better body mechanics and balance. Since the accident, I have learned to ski, scuba dive and live a very active lifestyle—I even grew an inch taller! I feel more confident that I will live longer. These are all benefits I wouldn't have realized had the accident not happened.

As I recovered, I often thought about the care experiences of ordinary people *without* the extensive medical knowledge or other advantages I had. Working on care coordination and health improvement at

AARP Services, Inc. puts me in a unique position to share my experience. After all, that car hit *me*. *I* now have an opportunity to speak up about it in a very public way and advance the conversation about how care should be delivered.

Resilience has allowed me to see how much good can come out of even the most trying circumstances. It allowed me to turn a disability into an asset, from a cane representing frailty to embracing my inner self who happens to have a cane.

I took away from the experience invaluable lessons and have a new outlook that I believe is in step with the foundational values of AARP. My experience—and my attitude to find a "new normal"—reinforces a basic tenet of AARP: to embrace possibilities throughout our lives, even during difficult times.

The Opportunity for Technology to Transform Healthcare

With AARP's tremendous expertise and insights into the older adult consumer, and together with national healthcare players, we believe that together we can transform healthcare more than any one entity could. This excites me because it creates the best opportunity of all: supporting the view of the consumer, and embracing a consumer-driven model of healthcare.

This means working with healthcare partners to a provide consumers with cost-effective and easy-to-use tools they can use to live well every day. It also means working with health professionals to change the way they present these options to their patients—moving from talking about what a patient "should do" to working with patients to help them understand "how to" use emerging technology to improve their lives. When we put patients at the center, we create the opportunity to do a much better job of understanding their life-stage, their perspective and where they are on their journey in life. It presents us with the opportunity to change the dialogue by asking not what's the matter, but what matters to you?

So, when my dear colleague Joe Kvedar kindly offered me the privilege and honor to write the Foreword to his book on aging and technology, I was excited—it is time to address age and reframe how we think about "What is Old?" Technology offers the chance to reframe aging by connecting us with the vibrant sense of self we all believe in and want to maintain no matter our age.

Each of us gets excited and delighted when we encounter the next big innovation in technology—the "gee whiz" pop of novelty. But for technology to wildly succeed in the space of aging, it is not that we become enamored of technology, but rather that technology becomes enamored of aging and of us. In reality, when it comes to aging, isn't technology the bridge that allows us to move from where we are today to where we want to be tomorrow?

For technology to succeed, three critical elements must be addressed:

Technology should be designed for everybody. Think of curb cutouts that were designed for those with disabilities, and are equally appreciated by parents with strollers and teenagers on crutches. Levers and buttons that work for 83-year-olds should work equally well for 3-year-olds. Instead of carving out the aged, we should be including the aging. We should be tapping into our older customers' experience and wisdom to co-design what will delight them.

Next, technology should reduce the burden of care at work, at home and at play. Technology can transform the way we make an appointment with our doctor, pick up a prescription and monitor risks in the home, unobtrusively. It's not just about using technology to improve workflow in a healthcare setting, but improving the workflow of life, such that we spend less time on the processes of healthy behavior and more time living healthy.

Finally, technology should create meaningful connections—to self, to others, to the community. Fitness trackers are the latest example of how technology can improve how we track our activity, our actions, and provide insights about our behavior to drive personal success. But technology should also facilitate building our social networks, allow us to be active with family, friends and colleagues, and connect us with our professional caregivers—eliminating our fear of being a burden on others.

It's not really about whether or not we should be embracing technology, but whether or not technology is embracing us, whatever our age. If we can use technology to keep our minds active as we age, bring social connectedness that is meaningful and results in creating purpose each and every day, we will have done much to transform aging and enhance longevity.

Here is the true opportunity of technology—to keep us engaged, productive and connected. In short, to assure we always have something to get us up in the morning, someone to share our life with, and with a smile on our face.

And why not work together to do this now? After all, "old" is life itself, full of experience, wisdom, acceptance and endless stories to share. The one universal truth we all know about aging is that each one of us is getting older every minute of every day. (I can promise you won't be any younger by the time you finish this book!) So, it's not theoretical. It's a very real opportunity, for each one of us to demand that technology helps us age well and take advantage of the years we now have.

Technology that supports meaning in life across all stages of our lives, capturing a daily life of love, laughter and legacy, will be the technology that succeeds. This book makes clear that technology can inform a vision of vitality we can all embrace: No longer will we talk about "Aging in Place," but rather celebrate "Thriving in Motion."

Introduction

When I was approached by my team to write a book on aging and technology, my first reaction was, "I'm certainly interested in the topic, but I'm not a geriatrician or an 'expert' on aging." And then I realized that I have been deeply involved in delivering healthcare to older people for more than two decades, not only in my clinical practice but also in my role as founder of Partners Connected Health. And I, like everyone else, am experiencing this aging phenomenon firsthand—as both a baby boomer who just turned 60 and as a caregiver, not long ago, for my father who had Alzheimer's disease.

The reality is, there is no separate healthcare system for older adults: It serves people of all ages, from all walks of life. Much of what we have been working on at Partners Connected Health is being utilized by older adults and has made a positive impact on their health and their lives.

But we have a lot more work to do. We have barely scratched the surface in terms of creating the kind of seamless, responsive and efficient healthcare system that is required for today's problems. At the time of this writing, our country is in the midst of a debate over the kind of healthcare system we need and how to pay for it. If everyone stayed young and healthy, we probably would not be having this debate. But the population is aging, and not everyone is aging well. We are also in the midst of a serious health crisis—the chronic disease epidemic that is afflicting all age groups, but especially older adults. And that alone has the potential to overwhelm the healthcare system.

The traditional way of delivering healthcare—face-to-face and in-person—is not working for chronic disease. Conditions like Type 2 diabetes, lung disorders like chronic obstructive pulmonary disease (COPD), and arthritis typically require changes in lifestyle and careful management to avoid complications. And the "see you in three months" follow-up is not serving the needs of either younger people or older ones. The fact that more and more older adults are requiring healthcare is forcing us to re-examine how we've been doing business and, in particular, how we can retool healthcare to better meet the needs of the ever-growing older population.

Since 1994, Partners Connected Health has focused on developing a radical new way to deliver healthcare and inspire wellness. That was around the time that large academic health systems, like Partners HealthCare, were beginning to feel the strain of managed care and restrictions placed upon providers. There was tremendous pressure to cut costs and improve efficiency, much like there is today, except we lacked the tools back then to do it effectively or without compromising quality. It was apparent, though, that the healthcare system lacked the resources and the infrastructure to properly care for the record numbers of older adults projected for the future.

We realized early on that the one-to-one, face-to-face, in-person, on-site method of delivering care was becoming unsustainable. Technology was on our side. The advent of the Internet, digital cameras, biometric sensors, smartphones, Bluetooth and the like have enabled us to design programs that extend our reach into the homes of our patients, or even around the world to consult with experts who can provide second opinions. Over the past 20-plus years, we have developed programs like Connected Cardiac Care, a remote monitoring program for congestive heart failure, and our suite of

"Connect" programs that allow us to monitor patients with high blood pressure and diabetes in their homes.

Back when we began, even the most forward-thinking of us could not have foreseen how deeply ingrained technology would become in the everyday lives of people—and how quickly. Now, nearly *every* object can become "smart"—that is capture, receive and share data via a vast, interconnected global network linked together by inexpensive sensors. At Partners Connected Health, we've coined a term for this phenomenon: the Internet of Healthy Things, or IoHT. In 2015, we published *The Internet of Healthy Things*, a book that focuses on the seemingly unlimited implications of technologies that enable us to monitor people in real time and deliver real-time advice and intervention. I am certain that the day when we'll see easy-to-use, engaging, intuitive connected health technologies that will inspire older individuals to a state of better health is not far off.

When I first started on this journey, it wasn't just about the bottom line. I envisioned a healthcare system that would enable physicians to make a more powerful impact on the health of their patients than was possible within the confines of a brief visit once or twice yearly. I also believed that technologies like home computers, cell phones and the then-early Internet would evolve to support a healthcare system where consumers could get care anywhere, anytime at *their* convenience. I also came to imagine a healthcare system that would become a more meaningful part of people's lives, to help them stay well and better manage their chronic conditions.

This new model of healthcare requires a shift in our thinking. In healthcare we've long thought that all of the work and responsibility is with the patient—that the doctor guides and the patient "complies."

With the growth of Internet of Healthy Things and connected health in general comes a new model of *healthcare delivery* as well. We now talk about inspiring patients to better care for themselves while integrating their wisdom, personal preferences and motivation into the process. Likewise, individuals as they age don't need to be passive recipients of help and care, but can add value back.

This book is about new connected health technologies that can enable older adults to better maintain their health and wellness. But the innovations in healthcare that I highlight in this book will not just improve healthcare for older folks. They will create a better and more responsive healthcare system for everyone.

Come join us in the journey as we describe how we'll get there.

—Joe Kvedar, MD
Vice President, Connected Health
Partners HealthCare

CHAPTER 1

A New Kind of Old

A book on technology and aging conjures up images of smart homes embedded with sensors tracking every breath and brain wave; empathetic social robots whisking older folks around town in driverless cars and 3-D printers spitting out replacement organs on demand. Yes, this book is filled with stories of innovations in connected health and the people behind them. It will take you to the academic and medical centers, established companies and startups where these ideas are being hatched, supported and implemented.

Although some of the technologies highlighted in this book may seem a bit futuristic, we are moving at a stunningly fast pace. If these tools and services are not already in use (and many are), they soon will find their way into your home and your life. And they will have a major impact on how you and your loved ones experience your later years.

But first, I want to talk about something equally, if not even more, important: How we as individuals—and as a society—*feel* about aging. Our attitude toward aging informs *everything* that we do. It influences whether we focus solely on the negative or strive to enhance the positive. It determines how and where we invest our resources; whom we include and whom we may (unconsciously) decide to exclude. And our gut feelings toward aging and the aged will undoubtedly determine how much we try to impose our own views about what we *think* is good for older people, as opposed to giving them autonomy and real choices. It influences the kinds of technology we design for older adults.

Today, the average life expectancy in the United States is 78.8 years, more than 25 years longer than it was less than a century ago. We have created a new stage of life, *a new kind of old,* a quarter-century of "bonus years" that have the potential to be active and fulfilling for individuals. By 2050, there will be two billion people worldwide over the age of 60, up from 900 million in 2015. Hence, there is a dire need for technologies and tools that enable older people to maintain their health and wellness and remain physically and mentally active. But it has to be the right technology that addresses the needs of this population, not what technologists and app developers think people want, but what older folks actually find to be both useful and empowering.

When it comes to our perceptions of aging, many of us—especially the young—are clinging to outmoded ideas that no longer reflect the reality of the twenty-first century. When I was growing up in the 1960s and 1970s, retirement at age 65 was very much the norm. We treated people over 65 differently and they in kind acted "old." It was the rare 60- or 70-year-old who went to the gym, participated in a charity walkathon, trained for a marathon or started a new job or even a business—activities that 60- and 70-year olds are routinely engaging in now. Back then, turning 65 meant you were over the hill.

I admit I carried some of these negative attitudes toward aging into my young adulthood. I went through a stage when I placed a high premium on risk taking and boldness, and I believed that anyone "old" was calcified in their thinking. Now I feel the opposite: I value the wisdom and experience of older folks and am a bit more wary of risk taking and boldness. I now recognize ageism for what it is—a prejudice based on preconceived notions.

Ageism in Action

The basis of ageism is that once you reach a "certain age"—somewhere around 60—you start to become physically and mentally feeble. Our society has a tendency to lump everyone 60-plus into a single category—they are "old." When the culture assumes certain things about people, we treat them differently. We become blind to their individuality, preferences and different levels of competency. On the upside, if we think people are weak and helpless, we care for them, tend to their needs and go out of our way to be gentle or kind to them. On the downside, we dismiss them and exclude them from decision making or as active participants in anything. In other words, despite their experience, we have low expectations about what they can do.

That said, our negative stereotypes about aging are starting to change, not as fast as they should, but we're heading in the right direction. For one thing, turning 65 isn't what it used to be. It no longer means retiring from either a job or from life.

Is my attitude "adjustment" due to the fact that I recently celebrated my 60th birthday? I appreciate the irony, but I don't think so. Rather it is a combination of things. I was at a conference on aging recently and one of the participants said, "We don't go to retirement parties; we celebrate transitions." As that attitude permeates the populace, 60 really *is* becoming the new 40. This new way of thinking combines synergistically with the wisdom that experience brings to give us a new cadre of productive, wise individuals with much to contribute to society.

The reality is, less than a century ago turning 60 was viewed in an entirely different light. In 1935, when the Social Security Act designated 65 as the age when people could begin collecting benefits, the average life expectancy was just 62 years old. The basic lifesaving medical interventions we take for granted today—like antibiotics, antihypertensive drugs and routine vaccines against diseases like polio, measles, mumps and rubella—were nonexistent. There was no preventive screening for cancer or heart disease. There was little known about the underlying biological mechanisms of common diseases such as coronary artery disease (CAD) and cancer, or the risks involved in smoking cigarettes, or the physical impact of emotional stress. Back in the early decades of the twentieth century, the notion that you were embarking on a new and potentially rewarding stage of life in your 60s would have seemed far-fetched if not outlandish.

Modern medicine has made enormous strides since the 1930s in terms of defeating common illnesses and extending the lifespan. Today, we can confidently expect that the numbers of the "new old" will continue to grow. By 2030, 20% of the US population will be 65 or over. As the population has grown older, our norms and expectations about getting older have changed greatly. In parallel, the opportunities that technology provides us have changed dramatically too. *This book is about these two phenomena, how they relate and how they magnify one another.*

Having a Purpose

I see mostly folks over age 65 in my practice and they are far from being over the hill. Many are still employed (about 20% of people over 65 are still working) or are active in other ways, either playing sports, doing volunteer work, serving on boards or taking care of grandchildren. I'm the first to admit that it's not just better medicine that is keeping these people vital and strong. Anecdotally, I see evidence every day of how important it is to keep mentally and physically active and socially connected as we grow older. And there is mounting scientific evidence that people with a purpose in life, who are engaged in the world and have a reason to get up in the morning, not only live longer lives but *healthier* lives as well. It is also better for society: Happier, more engaged older folks translate into lower healthcare costs and shorter and fewer hospital stays. That's not my opinion, it's a fact, and I'll talk more about the studies that prove it throughout the pages in this book.

Yes, older adults want to feel independent and empowered. Most do not see themselves as passive and helpless, lying on the floor waiting to be rescued by a relative who is monitoring their every move via their smartphone. They want technologies that help them remain vibrant or overcome any physical or mental challenges that may occur as part of the aging process. They also want to be respected for the skills they bring to the table. Wisdom. Perspective. Generosity. These are traits that can move society forward, in a good direction.

So let me dispel some myths that you may be harboring about older people. First and foremost, all "old" people are not the same, any more than all young or middle-aged people are the same. There is a wide diversity among *seniors,* a word used to describe pretty much everyone aged 65 and over, but it doesn't take into account that everyone is not the same. A vigorous 65-year-old is going to be very different—and have very different needs—than a frail 85- or 90-year-old who may be burdened with multiple diseases. The 65-year-old will be interested in technologies and services that enable him to maintain that vigor. The 85-year-old would need more assistance in terms of managing her medical conditions and the everyday tasks of living. But that's not all. She would also need tools to help her navigate the world and stay involved and stimulated.

Second, all "old" people aren't pining for their youth! It may be difficult for younger people to understand, but studies show that people are actually less anxious and happier with their lives as they age. It's important to remember that people don't regard themselves as old or decrepit (as younger generations might believe) and that people still have dreams and aspirations well into their later decades. I think that with the prospect of extra decades ahead of them, this is even more prevalent today among older individuals. This new view of aging is even reflected in how people dress: Older people today look different than they did when I was a boy. They wear trendier clothes (actually spending more on luxury goods than millennials!). Many own mobile or smartphones, and they are the fastest growing demographic on Facebook.

Last, but not least, all older people are not technophobes! There's a "new kind" of older person turning 65 who is very different than his or her predecessors. Chances are, these younger baby boomers—who helped bring about the self-help revolution of the 1970s and 1980s and who have embraced smartphones, tablets and the like—will be receptive to trying new digital tools to maintain a good quality of life. In fact, they will likely expect technology to be a part of their "golden years."

According to a study by Accenture, 17% of Americans over the age of 65 use wearables to track fitness or other biometrics (like blood pressure), compared to 20% of Americans under 65 who wear trackers. That's not such a big difference between young and old. In the United States, there are 30 million Facebook users over the age of 55—baby boomers are the fastest growing demographic among social media users.

And while older folks may balk at having to pay a higher health insurance premium or copay, they appear to be willing to fork out billions of dollars on pills, potions and procedures to stave off the aging process.

Older consumers are fueling the sizzling hot global "anti-aging" market, which, according to Research and Markets, will reach $300 billion by 2020, much of that driven by baby boomers seeking new ways to look and feel young. I'd like to add an important caveat. The "new old" are not interested in clunky, big-number phones or tools designed specifically for "old people." They want what everybody else wants: sleek and attractive looking tools that don't scream "I'm old." But they also require devices that are well-designed for aging adults and that are effective and "seamless," requiring little fuss or bother.

Smartphone ownership is the one area where older people are falling behind: owning a smartphone drops off at age 65. As of 2016, 27% of people over 65 owned one—that figure represents an 8% increase since 2014. In contrast, 85% of 18- to 25-year-olds own a smartphone. Since so many health devices and apps are linked to smartphones, it limits their use among the older age group. This is a shame and we need to do something about it. From the perspective of mobile providers and communications companies, the aging population represents a potential and large new market. *Maybe it's time to get over "ageism" and design some products that appeal to this generation—and that includes better smartphones!*

A Movement around Better Design

Despite significant progress—especially among baby boomers—there is still a demonstrable age gap within the older population itself in how these technologies are being used to improve health. The people who could benefit the most from connected health technologies—the oldest and sickest among us—are not yet using them. I would argue that the reason these technologies have not gained traction among many older adults is not the fault of consumers, but rather can be attributed to poorly designed devices that fail to meet the needs of the market. I'll be talking a great deal more about this later. Given the fact that physical inactivity, cognitive deterioration and social isolation are among the most profound societal challenges facing us all as we grow older, it is imperative that we help close this gap.

For the first time in history, we can communicate with people in highly personalized ways at exactly the time when that communication is most impactful. When we apply this design philosophy to tools that enable people to stay more active mentally and physically as they get older, and more socially connected, there is enormous opportunity to improve quality of life. Further, by recognizing the sheer size of the boomer generation as we hit our high-maintenance healthcare years, this approach allows us to keep people healthier and happier without exponentially increasing the cost of caring for them. If we can leverage your smartphone and wearables to inspire you to improve your health, we don't have to pay someone in the healthcare system to do it.

In order to achieve widespread adoption of connected health tools, we're going to have to make them better. That's a fact. In most cases, product design for older adults is an embarrassment. Tech designers, mostly young, aren't exactly "older adult friendly." And, the companies they work for are often criticized for their lack of diversity and favoritism by hiring younger people and discarding older employees. Perhaps this is why most everything is designed for millennials. My point is not to judge or chide, but to point out that there may be a serious lack of understanding of the needs of older people. We need to ignite a whole movement around design for aging, one that inspires healthy living.

Most wearables are designed for engineers by engineers who are obsessed with tracking numbers, which is of little interest to most people. But there are a group of trailblazing companies that are venturing into the wearables market, designing inspiring products that provide insight into how we think and feel. These startups include Muse, Spire and Empactica. They are an offshoot of a growing body of science that is exploring the role of emotion and well-being in health.

Engagement and motivation are two other areas we must improve upon. Healthcare providers have few tools to promote adherence to treatment plans and lifestyle improvements. Basically, we try to scare you into compliance and can do so only in the context of an office visit. There is so much more we can achieve using technology to inspire better health. We have to incorporate the positive aspects of social networking and the sentinel effect (I am accountable to someone who cares) without the negative connotation (Big Brother is watching). People need to feel socially connected, but they don't want to feel spied upon.

Examples of this kind of too intrusive technology are the companies that sell motion sensors that you place around the house. A "sandwich generation" caregiver two states away can get a message when mom hasn't gotten of bed yet, or when she hasn't gone into the kitchen to make lunch. What a relief for the adult child to know that he will be notified when something is amiss with a parent. Surprise! Most aging parents hate these sensors because they feel spied upon and as if they are being treated like children.

With older comes wiser. We can't use technology that oversimplifies and belittles people. They are way smarter than that. And maybe we should be asking the older folks what they would like. That's a radical notion. The other side of this dilemma, however, is the powerful force of denial. How many times have we heard about adult children who pleaded with a parent to give up the car keys to no avail, only to have a tragic accident occur? Older people don't want to be belittled or spied upon, but there comes a time when we all need assistance and some of us may not be ready to embrace it. I have not seen a technology that can thread that needle with success.

Healthcare Anywhere, Anytime

It is a fact that as we grow older we use more healthcare resources. I see it in my practice every day. Older patients have so many more office visits, tests, procedures, hospital admissions and so on. A well-acknowledged problem is the alarming growth in healthcare costs, particularly in the developed world and, of course, in the United States. You can see where this is headed. If the only interaction or tool for health that we offer our citizens as they grow older is a visit to the doctor, we will both bankrupt our society and fail to deliver necessary care. The math doesn't work.

The population is aging and the corresponding demand for healthcare services can't be met by one-to-one visits with a healthcare provider, even if we double how many doctors and nurses we are training. That can't happen and, of course, it would just increase costs.

Connected health allows providers to have one-to-many interactions with their patients. Through wearables, mobile devices, video calls and the like, they can use software as a tool to care for their patients and save the office visit for the most complex issues and neediest individuals.

One example of this is the work Partners Connected Health has done with a Sudbury, Massachusetts, firm called iGetBetter, which uses a tablet and consumer wearables (like a scale and blood pressure cuff) for home monitoring of congestive heart failure (CHF). Their technology is a fraction of the cost of the big iron vendors. Originally, we worried that older folks would not take to the technology, but they did swimmingly. In fact, because collecting and transmitting data from blood pressure cuffs and weight scales is not technically difficult, we started with the lowest possible data plan for these patients. We found that most patients used that data up very quickly because they adopted the tablets for other tasks, such as streaming video. They adapted to the technology just fine!

In a similar vein, I often remark that Skype was one of the biggest boons to the current success of telemedicine. Not that we use Skype for clinical video communication—it is not secure enough. However, as tools like Skype and FaceTime are used more and more to communicate with adult children and grandchildren, the comfort level of having a video visit with a doctor also grows proportionately.

And, we need to keep in mind that a new generation of "young old" is in the pipeline. These are people in their late 50s and early 60s who may cross the threshold into "seniorhood" in the next few years. They are also the population that will not react well to being treated like children—either in how we design our programs or in the user instructions.

Reaching Out to the Underserved

One of the reasons that I am writing this book is to jumpstart a movement to design better health tech for the people who really need it—those much older adults who may not be as tech savvy or who have difficulty using digital tools due to physical or cognitive problems. Most everyone would like to maintain the health and vigor of youth well into old age. We can do our best, but there is a natural age-related decline that occurs despite our best efforts. Some of us, either due to unlucky genetics or a not-so-perfect lifestyle, may embark on our older years in poor physical or mental health. Sure, there are plenty of 80-year-olds who are in excellent health and who manage quite well on their own, and even a few exceptional 80-year-olds who can still run marathons and climb the Himalayas. But there are also a lot of folks at that age who, due to disease or frailty, may find it challenging to walk around the block or get up from a chair or navigate a tablet or smartphone.

The right technology can be a real boon for these individuals. It can help them remember to take their medication or eat properly, or encourage them to try be more active and track their conditions without forcing them to sit in a doctor's waiting room. Most importantly, it can keep their brains active and connect them to the outside world. We are simply not doing a good enough job making the connection with older folks who may not be as tech savvy, but who stand to benefit greatly with the right technology.

A research letter published in *The Journal of the American Medical Association (JAMA)* in August 2016 reviewed data from the *2011–2014* National Health and Aging Trends Study (NHATS), which surveyed "community dwelling" Medicare beneficiaries aged 65 and over.

Researchers evaluated the use of digital health among this group by assessing how often they used the Internet to fill prescriptions, contact a clinician, address insurance matters and research health conditions. In today's society, these are pretty basic tasks that I imagine many people do every day. Yet, based on this data, only 10% of adults surveyed are using technology for digital health purposes; and they are typically the wealthiest and best educated. One of the authors of the study concluded that, given the low use of these tools among older adults, ". . . present day digital health may not be the best approach to improving the health of seniors and reducing the costs associated with caring for this population." I half agree. The "present day" technology part is correct; we need to offer people far better and easier tools before we can expect widespread acceptance. But I reject the notion that just because people may not be tech savvy or well-educated, they should be excluded from the benefits of the twenty-first century. Rather, we need to do a better job in removing these barriers.

Smarter Together

When it comes to connected health, we are at the tender phase that organizational theorist and author Geoffrey A. Moore refers to as "crossing the chasm" in his book of that title. Early adopters are on board. The concepts of telehealth, patient engagement through mobile apps and wearables for health are now widespread and part of the general discourse. But how do we get to the phase of early majority adoption. I believe this requires partnerships that allow us to extend our message to larger and larger audiences.

The partnership between Partners Connected Health, the Healthcare Information and Management Systems Society (HIMSS) and the Personal Connected Health Alliance (PCHAlliance) helps us to achieve this goal in two important ways. One is the recent decision to combine our Connected Health Symposium with the PCHAlliance Connected Health Conference which, in the past, have taken place just weeks apart. This will enable us to get the message of Partners Connected Health to a bigger audience and, in doing so, inspire change in the way healthcare is delivered.

Our collaboration with Charlotte Yeh, MD, chief medical officer for AARP Services, Inc., is another way we are extending our reach to a new audience and tapping a new source of information. Charlotte is a long-time friend and we consider ourselves very fortunate to be able to have her as a collaborator on this book. Her framing language around aging is unique and has opened my eyes to the close relationship between social engagement and health. For example, she educated me about the negative health effects of isolation. She also provided a constant reminder that people want to live their lives, not pay attention to their illnesses. This, by the way, is something that health-tech designers need to remember! Charlotte has had a long-standing interest in how technology plays a role in solving these problems and her knowledge is incorporated throughout this book.

AARP is also in the midst of a number of exciting campaigns that are relevant to these issues, including Life Reimagined to "inspire you with a vision of what your future can look like" and Staying Sharp, its online interactive program to maintain brain health. AARP CEO Jo Ann Jenkins is on a mission to *Disrupt Aging*, the title of her 2016 book and of her keynote presentation at our 2016 Connected Health Symposium. In that respect, we are all on the same page.

Under Jenkins leadership, AARP and J.P. Morgan Asset Management launched the AARP Innovation Fund in 2015. It's a first-of-its-kind investment fund with approximately $40 million in assets, which provides capital to innovative companies focusing on improving the lives of people aged 50-plus. The fund focuses on three aspects of healthcare: Aging in place; convenience and access to healthcare, and preventive health.

We are also tapping the wisdom of Jody Holtzman, AARP's senior vice president of Market Innovation, who first coined the term *Longevity Economy*. The Longevity Economy is the 100-plus million people in the United States over age 50 who account for $7.6 trillion in annual economic activity. That number is expected to exceed $13.5 trillion by 2032. The point is, this is a very big market that contributes a great deal to society. It is in everyone's interest, old and young, to keep the eldest among us strong, contributing members of society.

The goal of this book is to educate readers about the power that technology can bring in helping us lead more active, healthier and more fulfilling lives as we get older. And I hope it inspires all of us to do a better job at connecting these tools to the people who need them the most.

◆ ◆ ◆

A GERIATRICIAN SPEAKS HIS MIND

Selling healthcare technology is challenging, and not just to consumers but also to physicians, nurses and other folks on the frontline of medicine. These are your toughest customers because they want to make sure that whatever they recommend to their patients is safe, useful and practical. They are not dazzled by bells and whistles—on the contrary, they are skeptical of much of today's technology. Yet they recognize the need for good technology that will improve the lives of their patients.

If our goal is to extend the healthspan, it's imperative that we encourage older adults to start using some of these health-tech tools to manage their health and stay well.

Studies have shown that patients are waiting for their doctors to recommend connected health tools before they will try them themselves. If you want to reach patients, you have to first convince doctors that your technology meets their high standards. So you better understand what physicians want and need for themselves and their patients.

No one articulates the point of view of the physician better than Bruce Leff, MD, director of The Center for Transformative Geriatric Research and professor of medicine at Johns Hopkins Medicine, both in Baltimore, Maryland. Below, are some of his insights on the state of technology.

Too Much Information

I get pitched stuff all the time, and the purveyors of all of these technologies are constantly telling me, "I can give you all of this information." I say, "Listen, I really don't want all that information." If I'm a consumer using it, I want this thing to solve a problem for me. If I'm a doctor who has a patient who's using it, I don't want to be notified for every beep. I only want to be notified when the information is sufficient enough to necessitate some sort of change in a care plan. I think when they're finished talking to me, they kind of shake their heads and say, "Ugh, what a Luddite." I think people are getting a little better at realizing some of this, but there's still a lot of this type of thing going on in the field. Understandably, it's a nascent field and a lot of folks are just getting started.

No, There Isn't "an App" for That

A lot of the Silicon Valley generation thinks that the solution for a host of problems is an app. If you just send someone a text message, you're going to solve the world's problems. Or if you can get an individual's dry cleaning delivered without the person having to go to the dry cleaning store, that's enough. They really don't understand the clinical issues, the clinical problems or the population that they are designing for when it comes to health. I think that's a gap.

I don't mean to come across as negative on tech. I do think there will be good tech in time, but it feels like we're still at the start of something. It feels like the use cases and problems have not been as well defined as they need to be by people who are working in the field.

A Sensor Isn't Always the Answer

Tech folks are enamored of sensors and technology. I don't think, in general, that people have really thought about the problems that they are truly trying to solve. I think the tech world underestimates the fact that when its tech is in someone's home, it will also have a labeling effect. People who come over will ask, "Oh, wow! Jack, what are all these sensors in your living room?" And Jack will answer, "Well, you know, I fall all the time." It could be very embarrassing for someone. If you're going to do this kind of thing, it needs to be invisible.

Privacy is still an important issue. Sometimes, people are willing to give it up in certain situations for a benefit. But I think a lot of people don't want to be watched when they're in the bathroom, right? I don't think people necessarily want to be watched by cameras that are forever examining their gait or examining their urine when it splashes into the toilet or monitoring how many times they're going to the refrigerator. I've heard this a lot from my patients; they feel that this kind of technology infantilizes them.

Simple and Seamless

One thing technology could do is to create better linkages between health and social systems that would be completely invisible to patients. For example, let's say that Patient X is on Medicaid and meets qualifications for SNAP (Supplemental Nutrition Assistance Program) for food assistance. The system would automatically enroll that patient to receive SNAP because most people who are eligible for it never get it and never get enrolled. That same technology would reach out to the patient and say, "Boy, did you know you qualify for this? Would you like chicken tonight or beef?" And maybe the food could even be delivered to the home. That doesn't necessarily require physiologic monitoring. That's a big data problem.

It's sort of pedestrian, but another very big problem is getting medications into the homes of people who need them. Most pharmacies do not deliver. Most drug plans are administered by prescription benefits managers who have very strict requirements on when they will refill a prescription—even for very crucial medicines. If you go to the pharmacy a day early, the pharmacist will tell you, "No. Sorry, I can't fill that until tomorrow." I can't even begin to tell you how much medication nonadherence is due to that particular issue.

Quite honestly, I think drones might be a fabulous thing, in terms of a technology that will be enabling, just by getting things to people's homes when they need them, exactly when they need them, so that if they're functionally impaired and can't get out of their homes, the medicine just shows up. The food shows up. The daughter doesn't have to take off half the day from work to go to the Rite Aid or the Costco or Walgreens to pick up the medicine or the meal. Connecting things like that, that kind of tech, would be terrific.

The Basics

One good use for sensors would be adjusting home lighting to the needs of patients over the course of a day, whether the sun shines or not. A lot of older people have visual impairments and lighting can make the real difference between tripping over something or not. Most people do not have good lighting in their homes. This may seem trivial but many of my patients with visual impairment say, "Oh, Dr. Leff, thank you for telling me to get some more lamps in my house with brighter bulbs. I can't tell you how much easier it is for me to get around now in the evenings." Light bulbs! That's Thomas Edison stuff!

It would be a great thing if there was good technology that could do home safety assessments. Right now, it has to be done by an occupational therapist or a nurse who comes to the home. For instance, there could be an app on a smartphone that would let someone walk around the house and take a video, and then some technology could analyze that and say, "These are the 10 things you should do to make your house safer to live in and reduce your risk of falls." And it would make a list of things, like fix that hole in the floor or get some banisters on that stairway, and then link to someone who can contract for those services at a reasonable price. That will really save lives. That will keep people from falling much more than any kind of gait analysis algorithms that people are running right now. That's really useful. That would be transformative. It doesn't require wiring up someone's house for $20,000."

A Place for Robots

Down the road, I guess robots will get better because, in theory, the AI supporting them will get better and better over time. I would love to see robots that could alleviate social isolation. Social isolation is truly an enormous problem that technology might help ameliorate, whether it's through social robots, which we're hearing a lot about lately, or creating virtual communities, where people can communicate better. There's a lot of data—at least a lot of big observational studies—that show that the more people are socially networked, the better their health outcomes. It would be interesting to see if you could test robots or tech that created virtual social networks and see what the effect of that would be on health outcomes. It would be some really, really cool research to do.

I would love to see robots that could perform or help people perform activities of daily living. That's what gets people into nursing homes. Helping someone bathe or take a shower or get up out of bed. Helping someone get dressed or change a diaper. Making sure there is food in the house. Those are really hard tasks. I suspect one day that'll happen, but that would be one that would really be helpful. A robot that could cook would be nice too.

One thing something like an Alexa might be very good at is listening to someone who's demented and repeats himself all day long. Unlike the spouse who hears the question 50 times a day, Alexa won't really mind if she hears it 50 times a day. Figuring out ways to use robots to help people with cognitive impairment age in place might be good. That's an interesting problem for AI and the people who do those kinds of things. That's probably a pretty hard engineering problem, but I'm sure someone is working on that now.

The Future: Hospital at Home

More than 20 years ago, we started the Hospital at Home program at Johns Hopkins. It's an option for some patients to receive acute hospital-level medical care in the home as an alternative to typical, traditional care in the acute hospital. There are definitely some people who can't be taken care of at home, but we think probably somewhere between a quarter and a third of all patients could.

Hospital at Home came out of the observation that older folks tend to be very vulnerable to the challenges of being in a hospital and vulnerable to iatrogenic injury and insult, whether that's decline in cognitive function, decline in physical function, falls, infections or adverse drug reactions. And that's just by virtue of the fact that, as we all age, our physiology becomes a bit more vulnerable.

One use case is doctors like me wanting to keep their patients out of a potentially harmful environment. The other is that, in my experience, it's not at all uncommon for someone who probably needs to be in a hospital to say, "I really don't want to go there because it's a pretty lousy hotel, and I'd really much rather be at home."

To date, it hasn't been a very high-tech venture, except to the extent that we're doing some things in homes that are typically done in hospitals, like IV antibiotics or fluids, x-rays and certain ultrasound tests, blood testing at home, that kind of point-of-care stuff.

There are some models of Hospital at Home that are trying to do a bit more to bring what I call a biometrically enhanced televideo, telemedicine construct to Hospital at Home, which is probably the better way to scale the model over time. I think that as those capabilities improve, as the behind-the-scenes algorithms for monitoring improve, it will probably enhance the ability of Hospital at Home to take care of sicker and sicker patients or a broader variety of diagnoses and patients.

CHAPTER 2

The Challenge—and Opportunity—of an Aging World

"For the first time in human history, people aged 65 and over will outnumber children under age 5. This crossing is just around the corner, before 2020. These two age groups will then continue to grow in opposite directions. By 2050, the proportion of the population aged 65 and older (15.6 percent) will be more than double that of children under age 5 (7.2 percent). This unique demographic phenomenon of the 'crossing' is unprecedented."
—FROM AN AGING WORLD: 2015;
UNITED STATES CENSUS BUREAU

"It's only in Washington that addressing the needs of over 100 million people is called an unaffordable cost and financial burden. In the private sector, addressing the needs of over 100 million people is called an opportunity. Depending on which door you walk through, the unaffordable cost and financial burden door versus the opportunity door, you get into completely different conversations, and one is backward looking and one is forward looking."
—JODY HOLTZMAN, SENIOR VICE PRESIDENT,
MARKET INNOVATION, AARP

What may be the greatest accomplishment of the twentieth century could be the major challenge—or opportunity—of the twenty-first. In the United States, over the past century, we have added 25 years to the human lifespan. If we play our cards right, most of us can look forward to a very long life.

It's not just happening in the United States—the aging of our population is a worldwide phenomenon. Low birth rates and a longer lifespan are causing a global demographic shift—people almost everywhere are living longer than ever. The pace of population aging may vary from country to country, but according to the World Health Organization (WHO), by 2020, for the first time in recorded history, the number of people on earth aged 65 plus will outnumber children younger than 5 years. By 2050, the number of people 65 plus is expected to triple to 1.5 billion, representing 16% of the world's population.

The ratio of young to old is rapidly shifting. Between now and 2030, 10,000 people will turn 65 every day and will account for 20% of the US population. The reality is, there will be tens of millions of older adults flooding Medicare and social services, accelerating a growing shortage of healthcare professionals and rising healthcare costs, while there will be a diminishing pool of employed people to pay for it.

No matter how you crunch the numbers, the cost of healthcare for older adults is daunting. Although they comprise just under 15% of the population, people over age 65 account for around 34% of total healthcare expenditures in the United States. Overall, Medicare spending has slowed down in recent years, thanks to reforms like bundled payments and other incentives that emphasize value over volume. Nevertheless, higher prescription costs, as well as the sheer numbers of older people entering the healthcare system, will contribute to a rise in spending over the next decade. As noted in "The Facts on Medicare Spending and Financing," a 2016 report by the Henry J. Kaiser Family Foundation,

"Medicare spending (that is, mandatory Medicare spending minus income from premiums and other offsetting receipts) is projected to increase from $591 billion in 2016 to $1.1 trillion in 2026, according to CBO [Congressional Budget Office]."

The fact is, we are not at all prepared to address the implications of caring for an aging population that will soon be twice the size of a younger demographic, both in the United States and around the world. We are still, in large part, floundering, trying to quickly cobble together policies and services to meet the needs of the diverse and growing older population.

There is a gap to be filled, not just in retooling healthcare organizations to better manage their older patients in and, more importantly, out of brick-and-mortar settings. We must also create ways for older adults to get the most out of their "bonus" years. It's in everyone's best interest to keep individuals active and vital for as long as possible, employed for as long as possible and useful and productive in other ways, even when they no longer work for money.

There is also a desperate need for both creative thinking and quick action to fill these unmet needs. That is where AARP's Jody Holtzman's "opportunity door" swings wide open. The demographic shift from young to old poses a once-in-a-millennium opportunity for smart entrepreneurs, investors, startups and existing companies to design the next generation of tools that enable older adults to live fully and well throughout their extended lifespan. Later, I will describe in further detail where these opportunities are and how they can be developed. But first, we need to understand the breadth and scope of the challenges facing all stakeholders; individuals, society and the healthcare system.

Older but Not Healthier

Everyone experiences some wear and tear with age. As time marches on, even the healthiest body loses some resilience. Joints wear, muscles atrophy, organs begin to peter out. Nearly everyone, from marathon runners and yoga devotees to health food fanatics will run into one or more of these challenges with time. There is a certain amount of inevitability to the fact that we use more healthcare services as we age. My intent is not to suggest that we should live in a fantasy world where technology will allow all of us to live as if we were 20 years old forever. However, right now, we lump it all in together—lifestyle-related illness with genetic inevitability with bad luck from infection or accident—and all are treated the same. Technology can help us with the lifestyle-related part, the preventive part. While this is the focus of much of the writing in the chapters ahead, it is in no way meant to discriminate against the inevitability of the age-related diminishing of physiologic capacity.

But the kinds of maladies that we are seeing today go well beyond the wear and tear of "normal" aging. While we've managed to add a quarter-century to our life expectancy, we have done a mediocre job extending the *healthspan*—that is, increasing the number of years that people stay in good mental and physical health. I'm talking about the epidemic of chronic, lifestyle-related disease. More than half of all Americans now have one or more chronic diseases and older people are especially hard hit. Today, more than one-third of adults over age 60 are obese and 25% are diabetic. Nearly two-thirds of men and women over 65 have high blood pressure. Three out of four adults aged 65 and over have multiple chronic conditions, including prediabetes, diabetes, high blood pressure, arthritis and lung disorders.

If not managed properly, these chronic illnesses can result in serious, if not life-threatening, ailments like stroke, heart attack, cancer and severe cognitive problems. Although some forms of mental decline, like mild forgetfulness, may be in the normal range, experts are predicting a dramatic uptick in serious cognitive disorders like Alzheimer's disease and other forms of dementia. According to a 2012 report "Dementia: A Public Health Priority" from the World Health Organization (WHO) and Alzheimer's Disease International (ADI), the number of people living with dementia worldwide is estimated to have been 35.6 million in 2010, and it is expected that the number will nearly double every 20 years, reaching 65.7 million in 2030 and 115.4 million in 2050. This not only poses a huge and expensive burden on society, but can also place an enormous strain on families. Like other chronic diseases, some forms of dementia are due to genetics, but much of it is also related to lifestyle.

We know that about 30% of an individual's health is due to genetics or just plain luck (as in the case of exposure to infection), but the other 70% is dependent on the environment in which we live, and much of that is in our own hands. Right now, we are concentrating too much on the 30% and neglecting the 70%. This is proving to be very costly in terms of both money and human suffering. In other words, we are lagging behind in prevention, taking aggressive action only after someone has shown symptoms and, even then, treating each disease episodically.

A Healthcare System in Turmoil

The core of the problem is that the antiquated healthcare system we operate under today is out of sync with what is currently needed—and has been for some time. Our healthcare system was structured with acute diseases and injuries in mind. To be fair, it produced the vaccines that triumphed over childhood diseases; created the antibiotics that saved people from pneumonia and tuberculosis and invented the surgical techniques that prevented countless numbers from dying in the operating room. If you have a broken leg that needs mending, or suffer a heart attack, odds are you will get excellent care at almost any emergency department in a good hospital.

I'm not knocking it. Our healthcare system has brought us to this point, where most people can look forward to living well into their 60s and beyond, something unheard of at the turn of the twentieth century. But a healthcare system that is focused on acute care is poorly matched with the needs of the people it is caring for today. We're not going to solve the healthspan problem until we bring the healthcare system into the twenty-first century. And that means changing how we do business.

At an annual cost of $9,000-plus per person, the United States spends twice as much on healthcare as any other developed country, but our population is far from the healthiest. Our healthcare system is fraught with waste, mismanagement and disappointing outcomes. There have been many attempts at reform: For more than two decades, the healthcare system has been undergoing tumultuous change, starting with the move from fee-for-service to new payment models like capitation, bundled payments and those that favor value-based care over volume. For those of you unfamiliar with the lingo, it means that payers, both public and private, were trying to break free from a model that forced them to compensate everyone along the supply chain for every consult, test and procedure. It is widely believed that fee-for-service contributed to the 20% to 30% of healthcare expenditures that is wasteful, particularly redundancies in care, overtreatment and excessively high margins for basic products and services. It makes sense; under that reimbursement model, that there are no incentives to keep costs down.

So to combat the skyrocketing cost of tests, procedures and hospital stays, public and private payers offered healthcare providers alternative reimbursement models that rewarded efficiency and penalized bad outcomes. These new payment models were accelerated under the Affordable Care Act (ACA). Even though the future of healthcare is uncertain, and there may be many different attempts at reform before we get it right, one thing is clear: What we can't do is throw more money at healthcare.

The future isn't in more hospital beds, nursing homes, medical tests and procedures. The United States already spends $3.35 trillion a year on healthcare. In fact, healthcare costs gobble up close to 18% of our gross domestic product (GDP). Given the fact that our population is one of the fattest, sickest and unhealthiest among other affluent countries, there is wide agreement that we're not getting our money's worth.

As noted earlier, the majority of health problems today are lifestyle-related chronic conditions that cannot be conquered by the modern marvels of medicine. Effective solutions for chronic disease, which often include behavioral components, require frequent, personalized interventions that affect patient actions outside of the healthcare setting—where lifestyle choices can have the most impact on health and well-being. A brief interaction with a physician or nurse every few months, reminding a patient to eat better, get more exercise and find better ways to manage stress, is pretty useless without continuous and meaningful follow-up.

More than 20 years ago, when we founded Partners Connected Health, we anticipated the demographic shift and realized that the current healthcare system was becoming too costly, inefficient and ineffective. We understood that we would require new solutions that moved healthcare delivery beyond the inefficient one-to-one interaction to one-to-many, while maintaining the highest-quality care.

Connected health tools, like digital therapeutics—technology-based solutions that have an impact on disease comparable to that of a drug—can be an effective method of enabling people to better manage chronic conditions. Further, as artificial intelligence (AI) moves forward, the digital devices that have become ubiquitous in our daily lives will study human life and behavior in real time, moment to moment, in ways never before possible. These devices will automatically share this knowledge with humans, providing much greater insight about the inner emotional state of ourselves and others. Combined with in-the-moment automated coaching, emotionally aware technology will create a boom in self-help. I provide a deeper look into several startups offering these kinds of services throughout this book.

These tools can be deployed in real time and at scale, and can do what conventional healthcare cannot: provide in-the-moment intervention and guidance. If done properly, connected health tools can help to keep people well and on track when they're outside of the doctor's office. That not only frees up the doctor and other medical personnel to attend to real emergencies or challenging patient needs, but increases efficiencies and, ultimately, can decrease the cost of care.

Half of all healthcare expenditures each year go to the sickest 5% of patients, who tend to be old and frail. So it would make sense to find better ways to identify the most vulnerable and provide care and intervention before these patients end up in the emergency department due to often avoidable episodes caused by lack of adherence to medication or unhealthy lifestyle choices. Data science and predictive analytics can help identify patterns of behavior that could indicate a potential problem down the road and intervene earlier, when it's more likely to make a positive difference in patient outcomes—and reduce costs.

A Hit on the Economy

Skyrocketing healthcare costs impact every sector of society, but especially the economy. Lately, there's been a great deal of discussion over how to keep and create jobs in the United States. I'm not an economist, but I can tell you that we're not going to come close to solving this problem until we deal with the high cost of healthcare.

I heard a recent speech by the CEO of a company, which really drove this point home. He noted: "Name the product, but whatever price you paid for something manufactured in America, the leading factor that drove up the cost of that product was healthcare expenses for the workers." For example, when you buy an American car, the biggest cost is not steel, but healthcare. Thus we have trouble competing with cars made in Japan, where healthcare is a fraction of the cost. American-made products are more expensive because US labor costs are more expensive and a significant part of those costs is healthcare. We need to get a handle on healthcare spending, but we need to do it without sacrificing quality.

Another part of the problem, as noted above, is that we are running out of employed, taxpaying bodies to pick up the tab. In 1965, when Medicare was founded, there were 5.4 Americans between the ages of 20 and 64 for every American over age 65. Today, it is around 4:1, and in 30 years that ratio will shrink to 2.6:1. Unless we change the fundamental way we offer healthcare, we can't print money fast enough, or grow the population quickly enough, to solve this impending crisis.

And even if we change how we fund healthcare, we are still going to run out of healthcare providers. Our current healthcare system, for the most part, still clings to the inefficient one-to-one, in-person service model. In that respect, healthcare is light years behind other industries, like retail and banking, which have moved to one-to-many models of service.

If you're shopping at Walmart or CVS, you have the option of using a self-checkout machine. When you want to get cash, unless you enjoy standing in long teller lines, you can opt for an ATM. If you shop online, you may interface with chatbots to identify your needs before being turned over to a human being, and the like. Healthcare has resisted these changes; but that will soon come to an end.

The Association of American Medical Colleges (AAMC) projects that, over the next 10 years, there will be a serious shortage of physicians, with the shortfall ranging from 61,700 to 94,700 MDs. There is also a growing shortage of geriatric specialists and nurses trained to work with an elderly population. According to the American Geriatrics Society (AGS), there are about 7,000 geriatricians in practice in the United States, and we would need to nearly double that number by 2030 in order to meet the needs of the older population, *if we continue to take the unidimensional view that the only way we can deliver healthcare is if two people meet one-to-one in the same physical space.*

There is also a shortage of caregivers, both paid and unpaid. By 2020, 117 million Americans will need some form of assistance, either from relatives or professionals. Based on current projections, there will be only 45 million caregivers to meet this growing need, creating a gap of more than 70 million individuals to care for our elderly. On top of that, among professional caregivers (home health aides, certified nursing assistants), there is an extraordinarily high turnover rate, about 50% a year.

Staying Vital and Employed

The healthcare system in particular stands to lose if it doesn't develop new tools and strategies to promote wellness. As pay for volume moves to pay for value, keeping the older adult population healthier and less likely to need medical services is the new value proposition.

Michael Birt, PhD, principal for the Seattle-based health consultancy Blue Triangle, asks, "How is it that someone like Diana Nyad, at age 64, became the first person to swim from Cuba to Florida without a shark cage, yet there are other 64-year-olds who can't even get up from a chair or, even worse, have already died?"

Birt feels the answer lies in a better understanding of the relationship between genotype and phenotype, or how an individual's genetics interplays with his or her environment. He foresees a day when body sensors and other connected health tools will help identify biomarkers to provide a blueprint for how our bodies respond, positively or negatively, to things that are happening around us, in the context of an individual's genetics. "This is the dream," he notes, "matching the physiological data we're getting from connected health devices to how you live your daily life, inside and outside, if you will."

Birt is the former director of the Biodesign Center for Sustainable Health at Arizona State University. Prior to that, he co-founded a leading US-Asia biomedical business development company; consulted for many of the world's leading healthcare, medical technology and consumer product companies; and is the founding executive director of the Pacific Health Summit. In 2003, he launched the Center for Health and Aging at the National Bureau of Asian Research (NBR), while serving as an affiliate investigator at the Fred Hutchinson Cancer Research Center in Seattle.

Earlier in his career, Birt lived and worked in Japan where nearly 27% of the total population is already over age 65. He notes that Japanese society has made significant changes to accommodate this new age group, from training social robots to assist people in their homes to changing supermarket design to make it more ergonomic for older bodies. He adds that the United States is lagging behind Japan in that respect and can look to that country as a model of how to reconfigure a society to accommodate a growing older population.

In Japan, an increasing number of older people are returning to work or staying on the job, and, Birt says, it's not just because of financial reasons. For one thing, they're needed in the workplace now that the younger population is dwindling. For another, there is intrinsic value in staying involved in the world and a clear correlation between being engaged in meaningful work and maintaining health.

But there's yet another compelling reason to keep people on the job: Birt notes that economists predict that the cost of caring for an aging, retired population will stifle economic growth, both in the United States and abroad, for decades to come. "To the extent that our society can rebalance toward helping older people stay engaged and employed and earn some money, then that could reverse that slow growth," he explains.

Investing in Health at Home

Michael Greeley is a co-founder and general partner at Flare Capital Partners, a venture capital firm focused on healthcare technology. Michael has been on the forefront of health-technology investing for at least a decade. He was investing in digital health companies before digital health was a category. In addition, his blogs and commentary are incisive and guide the industry. As he sees it, there is a dire need to accommodate the surge in older patients, but it has be done in a smart, cost-efficient way that doesn't add to existing infrastructure.

"Investments in healthcare technology have become an absolute imperative," Greeley says. "We need these tools more than ever to drive greater productivity. We're not going to triple the number of rooms in hospitals to offer more care. We need new models like telemedicine and other tools that bring health right into the home."

Greeley adds, "I believe, and I believe the system believes, the great frontier in healthcare right now is in the home. You can get into the home in a very profound but virtual way and provide Massachusetts General Hospital or Cleveland Clinic–like quality care via telehealth and other connected health models. The elderly, the infirm, those populations have a really hard time accessing, engaging and navigating the best healthcare systems we have. We can deliver it to them right into their homes."

When using telehealth and other connected health tools, Greeley notes that, "There can be a lot of triaging on the front line. More often than not, older adults don't come in when they need to, or they can't come in, and sometimes they come in for things that aren't that significant. If we move the front line from the emergency room to the home, there's a lot of care that can be delivered—appropriate care at a much lower cost in those settings. Much of the healthcare innovation we are witnessing involves novel care delivery models."

Greeley also notes that the move to home care "takes on many flavors." And it's not just about delivering healthcare in the home. It's also about getting people the proper care when they need it, wherever they may need it. For example, many older people find it difficult to travel to and from a doctor's appointment. If they are unable to drive themselves or travel on public transportation, it often means that a spouse or child must take time off from work to accompany them. In some cases, providers can book nonemergency medical transport for patients, or even give out cab vouchers, but this requires additional time and paperwork on the part of the provider. Very often, nonemergency medical transport needs to be booked hours if not days ahead of time, which is not useful for same-time or emergency visits and can also be quite costly.

That's where Greeley saw an opportunity. Flare Capital Partners recently seeded a company called Circulation, a Boston-based startup that has preferred access to the Uber API platform for nonemergency medical transport. In contrast to conventional transport, Circulation makes it possible to book a ride just like you would book Uber. It provides a platform that enables preselected Uber drivers to transport patients to and from their doctors' appointments, picking them up at their homes, at a reasonable rate (no surge pricing!). If a patient requires special assistance, like help navigating steps, or uses a wheelchair or a walker, the driver is alerted ahead of time.

Circulation is HIPAA compliant, meaning it complies with regulations regarding a patient's privacy, a task that Uber did not want to manage. The ride is arranged by the provider, who subscribes to the service and also picks up the tab. This is important, considering that in some medical practices, the no-show rate can be anywhere from 5% to 50%, a loss that can add up to hundreds of dollars per patient. Taking steps to reduce missed appointments for a relatively small fee makes economic sense. Circulation also sees great opportunity in the clinical trials space as well as other healthcare transport needs.

Today's innovation is easier transportation to appointments, but right behind it is technology and services that will bring the healthcare experience right into the patient's life. Circulation and companies like it are a bridge strategy until society-at-large becomes more comfortable with getting its healthcare delivered in a truly time-and-place-independent manner.

Greeley says he is also looking at companies that provide comprehensive services for family caregivers, including linking people to screened home-care workers, managing renewal of prescription and over-the-counter medicines and providing meal delivery service for older people who live alone. Although he has not yet invested in any of these "one-stop shopping" startups for caregivers, he thinks that they will fill the need for the growing number of caregivers who are overwhelmed by the responsibility of caring for older relatives as well as their own families. (In Chapter 8, we profile New York City–based Wellthy, a startup that is representative of this new model.)

Looking "Beyond Walls"

Greeley noted above that the "great frontier" in healthcare is the home, and Sarah Thomas would agree. Thomas is senior director of Global Innovation, Genesis Rehab Services/Genesis Healthcare, and the executive-in-residence and innovation fellow at Aging 2.0, a self-described "global innovation network on a mission to accelerate innovation to improve the lives of older adults around the world." The fact that Thomas has a background in occupational therapy, holding leadership positions in elder care for nearly 20 years, as well as almost 10 years of consulting experience for emerging technology companies and investors, is reflected in where she thinks the opportunities lie.

"We're looking 'beyond the walls,' shifting the model away from the confines of an institution to the home," says Thomas. "We're looking at keeping people healthy and engaged at home and/or receiving their care at home. I look at companies that are trying to solve a true need while respecting people's individual preferences and choices for healthy aging, and creating a digital approach to customization."

When Thomas drills down on what services will be required to keep people healthy at home, you can begin to see how great a challenge—or how big an opportunity—it will be to meet those needs. Thomas notes that helping people succeed at home and in their community is the goal of Vitality to You, a division of Genesis.

As she explains it, the services are quite comprehensive. "For example, we make sure individuals are able to access their external community environment. Can they get to a grocery store? Do they have safe transportation options? We have a driving rehabilitation program to ensure safety with community mobility and driving. Are they independent with their money management? Are they able to ensure that they have healthy, nutritious foods? Are they able to grocery shop? Attend the necessary medical appointments? Are they physically safe in doing so and cognitively intact and/or supported in order to safely navigate their community environment?"

At the same time, Thomas says there is an increased need for better monitoring of residents to their anticipate needs and reduce the risk of problems in brick-and-mortar settings, as well as to make sure that the needs of people living alone are met. Toward this end, Thomas feels that data collection and analytics are essential tools to learning more about people.

"We need to be collecting as much information from that individual as we can, so that we are all able to make informed decisions about that person's care, with the individual and the family, as well as with the person's extended care circle," she says. "We need tools that allow us to identify and understand changes of patterns of behavior so we can intervene early if there is a problem. We need to be able to provide support and services in all settings, including the home, and take a more preventive and wellness approach, rather than just a reactive healthcare approach."

Thomas echoes a refrain that I've been hearing from many people these days: There is a need for better communication across the healthcare ecosystem so that everyone who comes in contact with a patient, as well as the patient himself, has the right information at their fingertips. "We need better communication across that continuum, whether you are in a home environment, a skilled nursing environment or a hospital environment. We need platforms that enable communication across the patient's lifespan, from before that person may have an episode of illness to his final days, to ensure that the patient's records are accurate and complete, and also that the patient's wishes are being followed," she adds.

For example, Thomas cites one startup, vyncahealth.com, as moving a patient's healthcare directives across the entire health ecosystem, thus honoring the individual's preferences in the process. The company's stated mission is "to enable the seamless exchange of high value healthcare information across the continuum of care, and to enable best practices for advance care planning and end-of-life."

I find it both fascinating and a bit unsettling that advanced care planning has become so complex that there is a company devoted to this. But, it is complicated and a variety of other companies are springing up to help individuals navigate the very complex world of US healthcare. Sometimes what is needed are tools to simplify dizzying processes rather than technologies that, while well-meaning, add complexity.

Tying It All Together

To Daniel Kraft, MD, the ultimate challenge is creating a unifying platform for a very fragmented healthcare ecosystem with lots of moving parts—none of them particularly well-synced to each other. Kraft is chair for medicine at Singularity University and founder and chair of Exponential Medicine, a cross-disciplinary program that explores how rapidly advancing, convergent technologies can shape the future of healthcare. He is also advisor to several leading biomedical and digital health startups. Kraft sees the aging of the population as a catalyst to create a new "aging infrastructure" that leverages new health technologies to improve people's lives.

"People don't often realize how quickly artificial intelligence (AI) and robotics and other fields are coming together, and there may be great business opportunities to build the tools that can help folks, and that aren't fragmented," explains Kraft. "In the future, your smart connected home, with things like Amazon Echo or whatever it turns out to be, will remind you to refill your meds, or do that mind-training game, or prompt you to check in with your grandkids. It will know if you are at risk for falls and maybe even adjust the environment in your home to reduce that risk. Your hearing aid won't just be a hearing aid; it can also be your health coach or it could remind you of someone's name if you forget it. Right now, many of these things are still a bit fragmented and kludgy, but they'll become more integrated."

Your health data will also be integrated into the aging health infrastructure. "There will be a blending of connected devices, smart AI and personal genomics, including everything from microbiome to genome to proteome. When we have millions of people sequenced, we will understand what genes lead to, not just, let's say, cognitive issues like dementia, which we already know a fair amount about, but different forms of aging and the risk of everything from osteoporosis to cardiovascular disease," adds Kraft.

Once we have a more complete understanding of the relationship between genomics and lifestyle, we can practice what we now call "precision medicine." As Kraft explains, "I'm hoping, in 20 years, that my health regimen—let's not call it an anti-aging regimen per se—is tuned in to me, my physiology and my data. My physician and virtual coach will know what my base genomics is, what my last microbiome looked like, what my performance has been, whether it's in the gym or just being out in the world, based on data from the 20th Fitbit version 30.0— collected from whatever technologies we have at that point in time. Each one of us will have our own personalized guidance and coaching based on our data and preferences. And this isn't just for older people, it's for everybody. Whether someone is 20 years old and trying to get into shape or optimize his fitness, or someone in her 90s and wants to stay independent, either person can leverage this information to be their own personal health coach."

What will it take to get from where we are today to Dr. Kraft's world, where everything in our environment is geared to keeping us well and staving off chronic diseases that can age us prematurely?

It starts with a commitment, from society and the government, to invest in wellness. You can argue that value-based payments for healthcare are a tool to mitigate unnecessary costs on the delivery side, but there has been no real discussion of investments in wellness, except as public heath campaigns (e.g., education on smoking cessation) or employer-led investments. There is now enough data showing employer-based wellness programs can have a meaningful impact on wellness and that government investments in similar programs for Medicare and Medicaid recipients would be justified.

As soon as we clarify the marketplace for tools like my friend Daniel Kraft describes, they will take off. Right now, they are sold based on a weak sales proposition—pay me $1 today to save you $10 next week. An economic model that supports wellness and home health wholeheartedly will go a long way to moving this vision forward.

In the chapters that follow, we highlight companies and technologies that have walked through the "opportunity door" and are filling the void, creating a new model of delivering healthcare and promoting wellness to older adults and their families. These include:

Care.coach, a platform that features an interactive avatar to engage people in their homes—or in the hospital—to promote medication adherence, detect cognitive changes early on and keep an eye on patients who are prone to falls.

Rendever, an MIT spin-off offering a virtual reality (VR) experience for nursing home patients, as way to connect to the outside world.

OhmniLabs, a startup with a telepresence robot for elder care that enables an older person to stay in touch with his or her family or healthcare provider in real time.

Sonde Health, another MIT spin-off that uses voice-based technology to analyze health and the user's emotional state in real life, real time.

Hasbro's *Joy for All Companion Pet*, a dog or cat interactive companion pet with built-in sensors and speakers. For ages 5 and up, it is used for Alzheimer's patients and as a tool to relieve loneliness, a prime example of intergenerational thinking.

Catalia Health's *Mabu*, a kitchen counter robot designed to improve medication adherence that makes eye contact and tracks the emotional state of the user.

Affectiva, a leader in "emotion AI," the new science of training computers to read and understand human emotion.

Omada Health, which offers a digital curriculum based in part on the National Institutes of Health (NIH) groundbreaking National Diabetes Prevention Program (National DPP).

Iora Health, a "whole new operating system for healthcare" that is focusing on the needs of Medicare patients.

We are still grappling with the inevitable problems that will crop up with an aging population and that will require a more responsive healthcare system and other social services to help individuals live safely and well. There is, however, a big potential upside. Today's older population is wiser, wealthier and the most generous in history in terms of charitable giving and volunteer work. If we get this right, if we can harness the potential power of older people, we can emerge on the right side of the equation and become a smarter and stronger world.

◆ ◆ ◆

ALZHEIMER'S DISEASE: A NEW APPROACH

Our healthspan hasn't kept up with our lifespan—and the same can be said for our *brainspan*, the length of time that we maintain our full cognitive function. Today, 5.5 million Americans are living with Alzheimer's disease, the leading cause of dementia among older adults. But that's just the tip of the iceberg: That number is bound to skyrocket as the baby boomers enter their later decades. The longer you live, the greater the likelihood that you will get Alzheimer's; 40% of all people 85 and over will experience symptoms.

I know from firsthand experience how devastating Alzheimer's disease can be, both on the individuals who are affected by it and on their families. As I mentioned earlier, my father developed Alzheimer's disease in his 80s and lived with us for the last six months of his life. It is difficult to watch a loved one deteriorate, but what makes this disease all the more terrifying is the lack of a cure or effective treatments.

Of course, a disease as complicated as Alzheimer's requires a multifaceted approach, including new treatments to address cognitive and behavioral symptoms, as well as better preventive therapies and healthy lifestyle choices, such as physical activity and diet.

But first things first—we need to better understand the underlying mechanisms and impact of this disease.

There is controversy among the medical community as to the cause of Alzheimer's disease. There is general consensus, however, that the accumulation of beta-amyloid (sticky plaques of ß-amyloid protein, which form around neurons), tau protein, found inside brain cells, and neuroinflammation play a role in the disease process. But research on animal models has not been conclusive and, at times, has offered contradictory results. Recent clinical trials using drugs designed to halt or reverse the disease in Alzheimer's patients have been disappointing, to say the least. There is evidence that suggests that a healthy lifestyle, especially staying physically active and engaged in the world, can protect against Alzheimer's. All of this is cold comfort to patients and their families.

Yet, despite all the negatives, Rudolph E. Tanzi, PhD, a world-renowned researcher and innovator in the field of neurology, vice-chair of the Neurology Department and director of the Genetics and Aging Research Unit at Massachusetts General Hospital, and the Joseph P. and Rose F. Kennedy professor of Neurology at Harvard Medical School, uses a word rarely used in connection with Alzheimer's disease—*optimism.* Tanzi believes that we have learned from our mistakes and are poised to start making real progress.

Since 1982, Tanzi has been investigating the molecular and genetic causes of Alzheimer's disease. Early in his career, he co-discovered all three genes that cause early onset familial Alzheimer's disease, which accounts for 5% of all cases; later, as head of the Alzheimer's Genome Project, he identified several others. He developed the "'Metal Hypothesis of Alzheimer's Disease"' and was instrumental in inventing "Alzheimer's in a dish," a model of Alzheimer's disease produced from stem cells grown in the lab, which mimic human brain cells. Currently, he is developing a potent class of drugs called gamma-secretase modulators to prevent and treat Alzheimer's disease by blocking amyloid production, along with therapies aimed at targeting the genes CD33 and TREM2 to curb neuroinflammation.

Tanzi is the bestselling author of *Super Brain* (Harmony, 2012) and *Super Genes* (Harmony, 2015), and the upcoming *The Healing Self* (Harmony, 2018), all co-authored with Deepak Chopra, MD.

Below, Tanzi shares his vision for a new approach to preventing and treating Alzheimer's disease, and discusses why he uses the word optimism.

Based on research done in your lab and others, you say that we have gained a better understanding of the cause of this disease, and we can now begin to move forward. Can you explain why you feel this way?

Basically, for decades, we were debating whether amyloid plaques caused the disease—and some people are still debating that theory. Based on new information, I believe we can say with certainty that amyloid is the cause of the disease, just like HIV is the cause of AIDS, or aberrant cell division in neoplastic cells is the cause of cancer. In the past, we were making naive assumptions based on studies in mice: When we put Alzheimer's genes into mice, they did make amyloid, eventually got inflammation in the brain and got sick, but they didn't get the other main pathology, forming tangles.

Tangles are what initially kill neurons in Alzheimer's disease and the lack of tangles in mice was confusing. And the fact that mice didn't respond the way we believed they should is what has fueled the controversy. But human beings are not 150-pound mice—we needed a different way to study the disease process in humans.

When we moved away from studying mice, we began to get a better understanding of what was actually going on in the human brain. In our experiments—the so-called Alzheimer's in a dish—we take human stem cells and turn them into neurons. In our lab, we regrow them in a 3-D gel matrix to create a 3-D neurocell culture that mimics a human brain, which we call a mini-brain organoid. We have found that if we have human neurons expressing the Alzheimer's genes, growing in a matrix that mimics the brain, they will make amyloid plaques within five or six weeks. In a few more weeks, they will make tangles. If you stop the plaques with experimental drugs in those cultures, you also stop the tangles. In other words, you stop the disease process. That was proof of concept. This didn't work in mice because mice have a different set of genes for this purpose, but using the human brain organoids, we were able to show that amyloid plaques do cause tangles.

If you look at the more recent work on imaging from other labs, it's very clear that plaques precede symptoms and if you have an excess number of plaques, eventually the odds are very high you'll get Alzheimer's disease. To me, this says that you have to treat the plaques early on, long before somebody has symptoms because, by then, it could be too late.

Has our approach to Alzheimer's disease been too little, too late?

Yes. What was happening in clinical trials is akin to waiting until someone just had a heart attack or congestive heart failure and then saying, "Here, take Lipitor. We're going to make you better." Or waiting for a tiny tumor to grow into a two-inch tumor with organ failure before you prescribe a tumor suppressant drug. That's exactly what we're doing now in terms of Alzheimer's disease! It's absurd, absolutely absurd. People are going to look back someday and say, "They waited until people had symptoms of Alzheimer's disease before they treated them." It's going to look like the butchery of seventeenth- or eighteenth-century medicine.

We were treating amyloid in patients with symptoms. I like to say, from the Alzheimer's in a dish we've learned that amyloid is the match, the tangles are the brush fires, and you can live with tons of plaque and tangles in your brain if you don't have inflammation. If you can blow out the match early on and limit those brush fires, you can prevent inflammation and never let it turn into a forest fire. The goal is to keep things from getting to neural inflammation.

Are you saying that even people without symptoms should be screened for this disease so that we can begin prevention earlier?

That's exactly where I was going with this; we already do this for a number of different diseases. Depending on their risk factors, at a certain age, women are advised to get mammograms to check for breast cancer. After 50 years old, it's recommended that everyone have a colonoscopy—and a colonoscopy is not an easy procedure. I'm sure in the beginning when someone said, "You know, I think everybody after 50 should have a colonoscopy," the typical response was, "Oh, yeah, right. We're going to do a surgical procedure on everyone." You do what you have to do. Similarly, I think that all adults should have a PET scan to check for amyloid plaque. Right now, a PET scan costs a couple of thousand dollars, and that price will come down, and it's a much easier procedure than a colonoscopy!

I recommend that after 50 years old, everyone should get checked for amyloid deposits. If you have a family history, I would subtract 20 years from the earliest age of onset in your family and that's when you first should get checked. If you're clean, fine, then wait five or ten years, like a colonoscopy, and then get checked again. If you're in the upper percentile for amyloid plaque in your brain at 40, 50, or 60 years old, go back again in two years, three years, one year. Keep track of it. The only way this works is that you have a way to stop amyloid deposition and empower those people with something actionable upon the diagnosis. I believe that lifestyle changes can make a big difference, and I also believe that we will have a drug that does this within the next five to 10 years.

Right now, insurance companies don't cover amyloid PET scans because they're not so-called "actionable." Although I would argue that with lifestyle, there are many things you can kick into high gear that are actionable if you know you have excess plaque at 45 or 50 years old.

And eventually we will have blood tests for Alzheimer's, like we have blood tests for cholesterol.

Even though there is no drug available right now that can halt the disease process, you believe that having information about your risk factors could encourage people to make lifestyle interventions that could make a difference. Why do you think that and what are these interventions?

I think that most people need a kick in the pants. When it comes to a healthy lifestyle, the stick and the fear of the stick works better than just the carrot. If you find out at 50 years old that you're headed toward heart disease, or let's say you have excess plaque in your brain as compared to the next 50-year-old and you're headed potentially more toward Alzheimer's, it's important for people to know there are things they can do to help maintain brain health and reduce neural inflammation.

I use the acronym SHIELD. The "S" is for sleep; people need to sleep eight hours every night, because that's when you clean the brain of debris like plaque. "H" is for handle stress, as in managing stress. "I" is for interact, that is, socially engage with others. "E" is for exercise; if you're not going to the gym at least try to walk 8,000 steps per day. "L" is to keep learning new things—that's how you maintain your neuroplasticity. And "D" is eating a healthy diet: Stick with a Mediterranean-style diet and minimize the bad carbs, bad fats, red meat and so on. I think if you know that you're in trouble, then you're going to go with a bigger shield.

If you could create an app or tool that could help people follow an optimal lifestyle for their brain, what would it be?

I think if your phone, or an app, could be set, to automatically bug you during the day and say, "Are you planning on eight hours of sleep tonight?" or "This might be a good time to get up and walk around a bit. Did you get your 8,000 steps today?" or "Have you learned something new today?" It needs to be just like a nagging mom with lots of repetition all day long, and repetition leads to rewiring. This is what Madison Avenue is based on. If you have your phone just reminding you of the aspects of SHIELD all day long, you just might begin doing it. If you do something for 60 days in a row, it becomes a habit.

I also think that people who are at risk (or even if they're not) could benefit from meditation. We've seen great results on gene expression with meditation—we had a trial that we published that showed that.

You've also been studying the microbiome and the brain. Where's the connection?

The microbiome of the gut directly controls neuroinflammation in the brain through the gut-brain access. We recently published a paper with a group from Chicago showing that we could alter the microbiome in Alzheimer's mice and significantly alter the amount of plaque in the brain—so you can affect amyloid plaques in the brain with your gut.

This is important to know because right now, at least theoretically, it means you can affect amyloid plaques with the Mediterranean diet or a probiotic diet, which I recommend in the books that I've written with Deepak Chopra. A healthy gut microbiome means less inflammation.

For breakfast today, I had a big cup of kefir with strawberries. I'm getting my probiotics from the kefir and antioxidants from the strawberries. I think there are things you can do with diet, from anti-inflammatory foods, antioxidant foods, probiotic foods, and by avoiding excess bad carbs, bad fats, and processed foods. These are types of things you can really kick into high gear once you know you need to be careful.

When do you think that there will be effective drugs or other treatments to prevent or treat Alzheimer's disease?

If things go swimmingly, I think five years is not impossible and 10 years is reasonable. My donors and people I work with make fun of me. They say, "How long have you been saying five to 10 years?" But of course, we made mistakes. We were treating amyloid in patients with symptoms who already had the "forest fire," neural inflammation.

We'll need the right drug at the right time for the right patient. We will need to treat Alzheimer's disease back when the first plaques develop, and that could be 15 years before symptoms. That might also be the time when you treat tangles. If you have a full-blown Alzheimer's case with symptoms, we will have to start treating neural inflammation.

There are different drugs in development. I think it's reasonable to think that we might have BASE inhibitors soon (a new class of drugs that has been shown, at least in animal models, to inhibit beta-amyloid in the brain). Maybe my gamma-secretase modulator will work. I've been working on this drug for 17 years and we're going into trials this year. Maybe one of the antibodies in development will work. I really do believe that within the next decade, we will have some drugs that work.

Later, if we want to achieve a brain healthspan of 120 years to match a 120-year lifespan—who knows how long we will be living by the end of the next century—then you're going to have to customize treatments and drugs to what causes neural inflammation in people.

And we have 20 different Alzheimer's genes that affect neural inflammation: I found the first one, CD33, in 2008. Over time, everyone is going to get neural inflammation as they get older anyway. We will need to know what's causing neural inflammation in someone so that we can match that person to the right treatment.

In addition to adopting a healthy lifestyle to minimize neural inflammation, like the things I outline in SHIELD, we need to look at your genes to see which ones are contributing to neural inflammation and we're going to have precision-specific meds for your individual case. If the lifespan is 120 years old, you might start those drugs at 60 or 70 or 80 years old.

It is inspiring to hear the thoughts of a true leader in the field. It makes me wonder if we had known some of this when my dad was younger, whether it would have made a difference. He was, for his time, a health-oriented guy. But, somehow, the disease got him. I also wonder about getting serial PET scans before we have real treatments.

This is such an important field and such a critical component of the aging puzzle. I look forward to following along as researchers such as Dr. Tanzi uncover more of the pieces.

CHAPTER 3

The Chicken or the Egg?

"Connected health is a change in how you've been handling something for your entire life. I think of it in terms of human 'change management.' There are steps that are needed to move people along to the new paradigm. Some people will grasp it much quicker. But there's this huge cohort of people, many of them are older adults—like my own grandparents, or even my own parents—who use things to a point and then stop. Those individuals need to understand the benefits of connected health in laymen's terms, and what value they place on that."
—REENA SANGER, HEAD, DIGITAL AND
CONNECTED HEALTH, IPSOS HEALTHCARE

"There are too many misaligned interest groups. There have been improvements, but it's coming together very slowly. Remember, for every dollar you take out of the system, you take it out of somebody else's pocket from a revenue standpoint. Every dollar of savings is a dollar of somebody else's lost revenue. People don't like that. They don't sign up for that voluntarily."
—LISA SUENNEN, SENIOR MANAGING
DIRECTOR, HEALTHCARE, GE VENTURES AND
MANAGING PARTNER, VENTURE VALKYRIE

'm often asked to predict what the healthcare practice of the future will look like. I don't have a crystal ball that can see into the future, but I do know that there are certain changes that are inevitable or the healthcare system will become unsustainable.

As the population ages, there will be more people to care for than we can humanly manage without making significant changes to the system. We need to explore new ways to deliver healthcare outside of traditional settings and we need to shift the paradigm away from illness to prevention. We need to make care more convenient and accessible for people who want to stay in their homes, or who don't want to readjust their entire day to have a brief face-to-face with a doctor or nurse. And we need to free up doctors and nurses so that they can pay attention to the more serious cases that require more care.

The medical practice environment of the future will involve both face-to-face and digital components. It will have to because of the looming shortage of healthcare providers and the growing demand for services. Doctors will spend some part of each day in office-based interactions with patients who have complex health conditions and require a good deal of clinical experience, knowledge integration and emotional support. The rest of the day will be focused on digital care delivery. Some of it will be checking on their patient populations via various dashboards indicating how they are performing on a variety of quality measures. Some time may be spent in brief follow-up encounters with patients via video. A portion of their day may be spent on asynchronous messaging with patients and other providers. Software will queue up which patients need attention and only patients who have not succeeded in the recommended self-care options will pop up on the provider's radar. In this model, physician and practice compensation considers time and complexity of activity, as well as quality of results achieved and efficiency in getting there.

Now let me bring you back to the present reality. Today, only a small fraction of health is delivered in the form of virtual care: We are still on the ground floor in terms of adoption. For the most part, as I mentioned in the last chapter, healthcare is still stubbornly stuck in a one-to-one, face-to-face service model. Given the enormous pressures on care delivery—an aging population, the shortage of medical personnel and rising costs—there is little choice but to turn to connected health technologies to extend our reach.

What will it take to build the seamless, efficient healthcare system that I described above, which delivers high-quality care to consumers—anywhere, anytime—while enabling doctors to focus their efforts on the patients who really need help?

When it comes to connected health, we are stuck in "the chicken or the egg" phase. Nearly every discussion I have about connected health these days, whether it's with medical professionals or lay people, typically ends with "but *this* has to happen first…." "*This*" varies depending on whom I'm talking to: Doctors, payers, health-tech device manufacturers and patients all typically end the sentence a bit differently.

In this chapter, I cover some of the major concerns that must be addressed before connected health becomes the new paradigm for healthcare. Let me re-emphasize how important this is for us to solve if we are going to provide high-quality healthcare to the onslaught of aging boomers we'll see in the next decade. These concerns include:

- fear of the "new" and "unknown" on the part of all stakeholders;
- archaic payment models that are resistant to change;
- privacy concerns among patients and physicians;
- the lack of a "prescription model" for connected health tech;
- poorly designed "consumer hostile" technology;
- an entrenched medical culture.

These are not insurmountable problems. But before we can look ahead, we need to get a reading on where we are right now. According to the Ipsos 2017 Global Trends Survey on Connected Health, adoption of connected health has stalled at 21% of the US population for the past two years. You would think that the adoption of connected health would be rising steadily in the midst of an aging population that requires more healthcare, is in the midst of a chronic disease epidemic and is facing a shortage of health personnel. But that isn't happening. The early adopters—fitness enthusiasts and the tech savvy—may have gotten aboard, but it's clear that we are not reaching all the people who could really benefit from connected health technologies.

Based on the Ipsos survey, the primary reason people are using connected health is to "monitor/improve their exercise level," not to manage a specific health condition. The reality is, people who are already tracking their activity are probably healthier and more fitness-conscious than the general population.

But the fact that connected health isn't yet the norm doesn't mean that people are opposed to it. The same survey also found that 69% of people in the United States who were polled said they would use a connected health device or tool *if it was recommended by their doctor* as part of their treatment plan. Another 52% said they would use one *if their health insurance company recommended it.* The lack of enthusiastic endorsement from doctors and insurers is a major chicken or egg problem that I believe is inhibiting consumer adoption. This is an important conundrum and will be an ongoing thread in this chapter. You can see where this conundrum would be magnified with older folks, who traditionally look to their doctors for guidance.

An Ipsos survey conducted in 2015 (including a Type 2 diabetes case study) revealed another interesting fact: Some 51% of US doctors polled said they have recommended connected health devices to their patients, but over half (54%) admitted recommending health tracking to only 20% of their patients or fewer. Who are they excluding? In our experience, we often see doctors giving the technology to patients as a reward for being more engaged in their care; that is. offering the option of connected health to individuals they feel are already tech savvy.

This is a prime example of ageism, rooted in the fact that many of us, including physicians, have preconceived notions about older folks and their ability to cope with technology. It also points to another problem. Those patients who could benefit the most are sometimes hardest to convince to use the tools. Until those attitudes are recognized for what they are, the group that could benefit from health technology the most will be overlooked.

Reality Check

In 2016, I was a guest on *Nightside with Dan Rae*, a nationally syndicated late-night radio talk show on Boston's CBS affiliate station, WBZ. Rae's listeners are a good cross section of the public and their comments are a great reality check and barometer of what people really think about the future of healthcare.

I started the program by describing connected health and how "it's not about the technology, but about a better way to deliver care," and how it was more patient-centric, easier and more convenient. I talked about our home monitoring programs for congestive heart failure and how much of what is done in the doctor's office can be done just as well through telehealth. After I finished my introduction to connected health, Rae took questions and comments from listeners.

Two callers really made an impression on me because they were decidedly negative. The first was a healthcare consumer and the second a doctor. The consumer wondered if virtual visits and connected care were as good as seeing a doctor in person, face-to-face. She said she was worried that this new type of healthcare would damage the doctor-patient relationship. I can only imagine her fear—that when she is sick and in need of help, she will be dealing with a cold-hearted machine and not a human being. This is certainly not the first time I've heard this concern among patients. Given the fact that connected health is still an unknown quantity for most people, we need to do a better job of describing the benefits and quelling this anxiety.

What's interesting is that the other caller of note, the doctor, also voiced concern that virtual visits and other connected health tools would disrupt the patient-doctor relationship. He then went on to describe his frustration with a system that requires doctors to gather data about patients during their brief office interactions, which means that the doctor often has his back to the patient during an office visit. (So much for the "face-to-face" myth!)

I've heard this complaint numerous times before from patients and doctors, and it would be easy to dismiss these folks as tech-phobic or "Luddites." But the fact is, there are problems with technology that we need to both acknowledge and solve.

On the talk show my response to the negative callers was something to the effect of, "If we design it that way, we will have failed." Admittedly, my answer was rushed because the hour show was ending, but concerns about clunky or intrusive technology are important and need to be addressed. I do, in depth, later in this book.

But I'd like to get back to the concern of the caller who sounded very worried about the impact of connected health on her life. Reena Sanger, quoted earlier, hit the nail on the head when she said that, as face-to-face, in-person healthcare shifts to connected health, we're asking people to break with an old, familiar model and try something that must seem very different. We're giving individuals more responsibility for their health than they've had before. I think that is the primary reason why people are looking to their doctors and insurers to provide guidance on connected health tools—they need reassurance that their care will be as good, if not better, than what they already have.

Nowadays, we talk a lot about the consumerization of health and how people want to feel empowered, and that's true . . . to a point. I have found, especially among my older patients, that they want reassurances from their doctors that they are doing the right thing. So, if doctors are not recommending connected health tools, and if patients are not asking their providers for a recommendation, well, we have the classic chicken or egg dilemma. It's an illustrative—and vicious—cycle.

I've been a connected health evangelist for more than two decades and I've seen, firsthand, how connected health can improve healthcare delivery. I know that many people reading this book are also among the already converted. Typically, we meet up with other like-minded connected health cheerleaders at conferences and symposia and forget that there is a large percentage of the public that remains skeptical—or weary—of change. This is especially true in something as vital as healthcare.

Doctors have tremendous influence over their patients; as we see from the Ipsos survey mentioned above. And, as I have heard from numerous patients, many individuals will "cross the chasm" to connected health if their doctors lead the way. But doctors have their own concerns; their own list of "but this has to happen first."

What Worries Doctors

Based on their survey of 1,300 physicians, in September 2016, the American Medical Association (AMA) reported, "There is a sense of enthusiasm among physicians for digital health." According to this report, 85% of survey participants " . . . overwhelmingly see the potential for digital health to favorably impact patient care." I agree that, in theory, doctors recognize that connected health is a good thing. In practice, given the 21% adoption figure, we have a ways to go.

If you ask doctors if they recommend connected health solutions to their patients, many will say that they're waiting for consumers to ask about connected health before they mention it. They are also waiting for some other things to fall into place.

According to this AMA survey, "Physicians require digital tools to fit within their existing systems and practices." Specifically, physicians cited four elements essential for the adoption of digital health tools: (1) liability coverage, (2) data privacy, (3) workflow integration with electronic health records (EHRs) and (4) reimbursement-billing procedures. Finally, the AMA reports, "Physicians also look for tools that are easy to use and proven effective." I call this fifth point *validity of technology*. I go into all of these points, below.

Liability coverage This is a big concern, so let me tackle it first. I have found that some doctors are confused about their responsibility to a patient who is tracking herself 24/7. This is understandable, as this world is somewhat confusing and evolving. First, let's acknowledge that the risks are no different than in the face-to-face world. As doctors, we have a duty to put a patient's health first: We must adhere to the "standard of care." At the moment, the standard of care is taking your blood pressure in the office from time to time and making clinical decisions on that basis. It is unlikely a doctor will be sued for failing to implement home blood pressure monitoring because that exceeds the standard of care.

However, once I order home blood pressure monitoring, it is like ordering any other test. I need to either be looking at the readings myself or have another provider checking them. This is the part that worries doctors the most. Until we come up with software that is able to take home readings and cull their clinical meaning—and it must be clinically validated and approved by the US Food and Drug Administration (FDA)—this risk is best mitigated in two ways. First, we must educate patients that connected home monitoring is not a substitute for calling 911. We must educate them about what out-of-parameter readings mean and urge them to get medical help if their readings are persistently high or low. This is best done by a thorough informed consent process. Second, home monitoring programs work best in settings where a clinician (often a nurse or pharmacist) monitors the readings from time to time and can alert the physician to patterns that spell trouble brewing.

Doctors also worry that because the patient is not in front of them, they will miss some important diagnostic clue and be held liable for it later. We advise reminding patients that a physician's clinical decision making is based on the information at hand (and not on information the clinician doesn't know about). This type of risk is not new. Those of us covering for colleagues on off hours, who take phone calls from acutely ill patients, deal with this all the time. Clinical judgment comes into play: If a doctor thinks you should be seen in person, it is best to follow that advice.

Most malpractice carriers insure for telehealth these days. Doctors should have a dialogue with their carrier before getting involved and have thoughtful informed consent about the use of these tools.

Data privacy Physicians are also concerned about the privacy of patients, or more to the point, violating the HIPAA Privacy Rule, which can result in steep penalties and angry patients. They can't simply send out a casual text or email. All communication with patients has to comply with HIPAA, protecting individuals' medical records and other personal health information by using secure platforms. I also hear a great deal about privacy concerns from patients who are worried about who will have access to their data. I explore this issue more deeply in a box at the end of Chapter 4.

Workflow integration Another very legitimate provider concern is workflow. Between seeing patients every 10 minutes or so, filling out forms, updating EHRs and keeping up with his or her medical specialty, the typical doctor's day is jam-packed. Physicians don't want to be bombarded by emails or texts from patients. They don't have time to fit this in and in many cases (and this gets back to the chicken or the egg) do not have mechanisms in place to be compensated for time spent on these activities. Similarly, they don't fancy being overwhelmed by patients who expect them to review their Fitbit data every day!

Reimbursement-billing procedures As just noted, the reimbursement issue is a major stumbling block to adoption. The business model that will allow doctors to be compensated for this work is in its infancy. With rare exception, as I've noted multiple times, the system favors in-person care and has structured reimbursement models accordingly.

Medicare has made some strides in this area. The Medicare Chronic Care Management (CCM) program now compensates providers for care coordination and non-face-to-face care. One option for providers billing the CCM code is to use telehealth visits or remote monitoring to coordinate care for patients with two or more chronic medical conditions. They can also use nurse call lines and other tools. (The CCM codes are not telemedicine reimbursement codes.) But reimbursement for non-face-to-face interactions is still pretty limited.

To be honest, some of my colleagues may view connected health as an economic threat. The move to value-based payment encourages innovations that promote efficiency, but usually means that someone along the supply chain is losing out. The mere fact that a patient isn't on-site means that there will be fewer tests and procedures performed. That's money out of somebody's pocket.

Validity of technology For connected health to work, physicians have to be convinced of the validity of the technology before they become evangelists. As noted earlier, there are numerous reasons why doctors are reluctant to use connected health. Fear of liability is one of them. It's not just about the fear of being sued if something goes awry—I'm not saying that tort reform wouldn't help all aspects of healthcare—but it's not the only concern at play here. Rather, in this case, their uneasiness is similar to the anxiety many doctors feel when dealing with off-label treatments for cancers or other illnesses. They take their Hippocratic Oath seriously and worry they might harm someone by endorsing an unfamiliar treatment regimen or one that is unproven, especially when more standard treatments exist. Hence, they want more proof that connected health is a "best practice."

Furthermore, many physicians remain unconvinced that virtual care works as well as in-person encounters. There is a deep-seated notion that face-to-face care is superior. This may change as medical schools update their curricula to include digital health tools and younger, tech savvy doctors who grew up with smartphones replace older providers. Another answer is scientific validation of new technologies following the paradigm used in pharmaceuticals. This is something we have great experience with at Partners Connected Health. The upside is that clinical trials pave the way for clinician adoption. The downside is they take time and add to development costs. We continue to search for ways to speed up this critical validation process.

And as if all these concerns aren't enough, in an era of robots in the operating room, self-driving cars and IBM's Watson being tapped for diagnostic and treatment recommendations, I believe there is an almost visceral fear among physicians—and patients—that machines will replace human beings. As a doctor, I am certainly an advocate for using technology when it's appropriate, and I understand that artificial intelligence may help make healthcare more efficient and effective and extend our reach. But as a human being I know that no one wants to get a cancer diagnosis from an avatar or have a baby delivered by a machine.

The flip side is that in healthcare, all we offer you now is services delivered by people. We have to embrace the fact that machines can do some tasks better than people. Delegating information-heavy tasks to computers should free us up to deliver those aspects of service that machines cannot: emotional intelligence, caring and judgment.

Follow the Money

This brings us to the next chicken or egg conundrum. Many insurers are waiting for more clinical studies to show cost savings and/or better outcomes before they fully commit to connected health. AARP's Jody Holtzman predicts that payers will see the data first and take the lead on covering certain products and services. He explains, "They will be followed by CMS (Centers for Medicare & Medicaid Services), who will want more data, but one X-factor is how all of this will play out in the current political environment."

Holtzman adds, "It's going to take a while before there is enough data to confirm that narrative. I think the biggest challenge is quickly developing the data that confirms these technologies will result in better health outcomes, which will lead to lower cost to the system. Lower cost to the system writ large and lower cost to payers in particular. I think when health insurers can start seeing results and cost savings, and have a sufficient level of trustworthy data to prove it, there will be greater adoption."

A handful of companies are investing in clinical studies and are being rewarded for their efforts. In 2015, the Centers for Disease Control and Prevention (CDC) recognized digital programs—including one from Omada Health—as meeting the evidence-based standards for the agency's National Diabetes Prevention Program. In March 2016, Medicare began reimbursing CDC-recognized providers like Omada Health for administering the National Diabetes Prevention Program to older adults covered by Medicare or Medicaid.

Back in 2013, Palo Alto, California–based Glooko, Inc., founded in 2010, received FDA 510(k) clearance for its mobile solution for diabetes management. And in 2017, WellDoc, another diabetes management company, gained 510(k) Class II clearance for a nonprescription version of its BlueStar digital therapeutic platform from the FDA. Baltimore-based WellDoc was founded in 2005 by Suzanne Sysko Clough, MD, an endocrinologist, and her brother, Ryan Sysko. Both programs are used by many corporate wellness programs and healthcare systems and are reimbursed by several insurers.

To clarify one point: FDA "clearance" is different from FDA "approval." Class II devices are cleared for market via the 510(k) process, whereas Class III devices must undergo premarket approval. Devices that receive Class III premarket approval are deemed both safe and effective and the FDA ensures that the manufacturer has fully implemented the necessary procedures to meet the FDA's Quality Management System (QMS). These Class lll medical devices typically undergo more rigorous clinical evaluation than Class ll products.

According to Bradley Merrill Thompson, digital health and combination product regulatory attorney at Epstein Becker & Green, P.C., "A Class ll product is more like a generic drug; based on FDA review, it means that your product is *substantially equivalent* to products that are legally on the market."

Thompson notes that this may sound like legal hairsplitting, but it's not. According to Thompson, "The FDA gets very particular about this.

They won't let people with Class ll product clearance say, 'My product has been approved as safe and effective.' Similar to generic drugs, Class ll products are reviewed on a comparative basis to see whether your product functions the same as products that are lawfully on the market, which by the way, implicitly has a safety and effectiveness component to it. But it's not an affirmative FDA determination that your particular product is safe and effective."

Some other products are required to go through premarket review as well. As Thompson explains, "If your product is an accessory (either a software or a hardware accessory) to a medical device, then this is the case. This really comes into play where you're talking about a blood glucose meter, for example, which is a Class ll medical device. If you make a piece of hardware or software that accessorizes that medical device, then your product is FDA regulated and it needs to be cleared."

There's a side benefit to achieving Class ll clearance for a product. It gives doctors more confidence to prescribe it and it is more likely to be covered by a payer.

But most companies are not taking this route. That's because they are leery of the investment required to get FDA approval and because of the slow sales cycle for new programs and devices for the US healthcare market. To their way of thinking, it's foolish to invest time and money in studies if there is no guarantee that either payers or providers will buy in. Why should they bother if it is so much easier and profitable to sell fitness trackers and apps into the fitness market?

That leaves it up to the consumer, who has been programmed to believe that anything related to healthcare should be "covered" by somebody else. Admittedly, there are many roadblocks to overcome before connected health becomes so embedded in healthcare that we no longer need to use the term *connected health* to distinguish it from the "other" kind of health. It will be one in the same.

A Winning Reimbursement Model

I don't want to make your head spin any more than I have to, but this goes back to the question, "Why do the studies if there's no reimbursement model?" I have given a great deal of thought to what a viable option would look like and I imagine that a winning reimbursement model would mix the following variables:

- It would reward providers of all types, including hospitals, for a combination of effort, efficiency and outcomes. The formula would be created in such a way as to maximize efficiency without incurring negative outcomes.
- The human provider portion would define "work" more broadly than current reimbursement mechanisms (i.e., not just face-to-face time with patients). I envision a formula that takes into account time spent, quality generated and efficiency achieved. If this sounds like the famous resource-based relative value scale (RBRVS) that Medicare now uses to set physician reimbursements, it would in fact have some similarities. The RBRVS considers the amount of training and procedural skill required (complexity), time spent and office expense. It does not make mention of outcomes or quality. This is a fine framework to use as a starting place to value work done virtually.
- It would correct for the healthcare system's disproportionate reward for procedures.

Ideally, one of the input variables would be from patient feedback—not just satisfaction, but something more sophisticated like a "feeling cared for" index. We know that when patients feel cared for they tend to be more engaged with their care. This, in turn, leads to better outcomes.

And, once again, this is why I think that human practitioners will not become obsolete, replaced by artificial intelligence.

My version of a reimbursement model would also include some patient/consumer aspects as well. The "somebody else should pick up the tab no matter what I do" model of healthcare isn't working. If we now know that roughly 70% of health is due to lifestyle, we need to promote healthy behaviors.

We used to ask, half-jokingly, "Why not have pay-for-performance for patients?" Not such a bad idea! In my model, insurance premiums would be adjusted so that members exhibiting healthy behaviors— those who don't smoke, get enough exercise and try to maintain a good weight—would *pay less*. Those that abuse their health would not necessarily be punished, but the baseline premiums would be high. There would be no free services, but copays would be quite low for preventive services.

UnitedHealth Group is experimenting with its own version of "pay-for-performance for patients." The company recently launched a program called UnitedHealthcare Motion that lets members earn money for out-of-pocket medical expenses by walking. What started as a pilot in 12 states, Motion is now available in 40 states and includes access to additional customized activity trackers through a "bring-your-own-device" (BYOD) model. Fitbit's Charge2 is the newest activity tracker integrated into the BYOD model. Qualcomm Life's 2net Platform provides secure data transfer and enables the BYOD model to integrate more activity trackers.

Enrollees in Motion are encouraged to regularly meet three daily walking goals (as measured by the tracker) in order to earn up to $1,500 per year. The program's F.I.T. walking goals are based on the need to walk with Frequency (300 steps in 5 minutes at least 6 times a day, at least an hour apart), Intensity (a walk of 3,000 steps within 30 minutes once a day) and Tenacity (10,000 total steps per day).

As with any health-insurer model, this program is offered in collaboration with the enrollee's employer. Employers can achieve a goal of a 6% premium cap if they achieve 60% compliance across all three walking goals among their employees. Motion is available to small, self-funded employers and large companies with fully insured health plans.

To sum up, some of the pieces needed to create a "new and improved" mode of reimbursement for connected health are in place. However, there are still few examples of digital tools that have the same impact on disease in the way pharmaceuticals do. This is where building the evidence base comes in (although evidence is growing, it is still scant). The second challenge is that the business model does not yet exist that would prompt payers to cover prescribed devices and apps, presumably at a higher price than they'd pay for consumer-grade devices and apps.

Design for Failure

Even if all the pieces fall into place and the developers, providers, regulators and insurers all get their ducks (or chickens?) in a row, there's yet another roadblock to widespread adoption: poor patient adoption. One of the reasons for this is poor design. Even if doctors could write prescriptions for connected health devices, I doubt that most patients would use them unless the technology fit easily into their lives.

In Chapter 1, I highlighted the need for movement around designing better technology for everybody—but especially for older adults. When I describe good technology, I use the words *seamless, effortless* and *intuitive,* but for the most part, today's health tech is anything but.

Unless we make an effort to correct what I earlier called "poorly designed 'consumer hostile' technology," we will never achieve widespread adoption, especially among a group that may not be as willing to put up with design flaws as younger users. Dennis Lally is co-founder of Rendever, a virtual reality platform built to improve the aging process for older adults by providing cognitive stimulation and therapeutic virtual experiences. Rendever's platform was designed with the older adult in mind and Lally feels strongly that more product designers need to follow the company's example. In "Why Tech Firms Can't Ignore Seniors," posted on *fortune.com*, Lally wrote, " . . . younger designers often have their own expectations of how seniors should think or act, and don't truly understand their needs. As a result, new tech products often fail to catch on with seniors." Lally also pointed out that the "design-for-all" school of thought doesn't take into account that older adults may require some modifications in design, including "larger fonts, increased color contrast and louder audio or subtitles."

Rendever is a spin-off from the MIT Sloan School of Management, where Lally completed his MBA studies. When we followed up with Lally, he noted that despite preconceived notions that older people are technology adverse, the truth is, based on recent studies, 59% of people over 65 are on the Internet. Lally believes that older people are willing to try new technologies, but not willing to stick with them if they don't work right away. "For my generation, if a technology's not great, we'll give it another shot, because we've grown up doing that," he explains. "But when older people try a new technology and it doesn't work well right away, they get discouraged. They think, 'Oh, I failed, I'm not going to try it again.' It's really up to the designer to build a product that they're willing to try, and that works from the get-go." I agree with these sentiments.

Another observation is that people don't want to work with "sad" technology that reminds them that they are "sick." Here's another tip for developers: Try to make your devices more like "cool" gadgets than something you would find in a sickroom. Our designers focus on designing for trust and empathy and on features that make software relevant to your everyday life.

It's true that older Americans may not be as comfortable with technology as digital natives who grew up with tablets and smartphones and who are accustomed to maintaining virtual relationships. Unlike our kids or grandkids, we don't think it's perfectly natural to conduct our interactions with other human beings in a virtual context. If you're of a certain generation, this stuff is unfamiliar. I've even noticed that older patients reflexively think that contact with a human being is better. Some of the initial reluctance to deal with virtual interactions may be due to the newness of technology, but I also believe it's because we haven't provided any good role models.

There was a moment at the 2016 PCHAlliance Connected Health Conference that underscored the need for a major upgrade in health tech, to enable universal plug-and-play connectivity. During the Q&A session for the "Connected Caregiving" panel, moderated by AARP's Jody Holtzman, a young man stepped up to the microphone and identified himself as a nurse. He said that when he worked with family members caring for an aged or ill relative, he tried to steer them to digital health tools that he thought they would find useful. But very often they didn't even want to hear about it. They would explain that they were so overwhelmed, they couldn't bear the thought of having "one more thing to do."

While this may sound like an easy excuse—that people just don't want to be bothered—it's actually an important statement that we also frequently hear from doctors. When people are overwhelmed, overburdened or overworked, the last thing they want is something they perceive can add complexity, more work or stress.

Says Holtzman, "The only way I see getting beyond the current hurdle of having to learn something new is when the simplicity of the technology doesn't require you to learn, when the technology has been designed to adapt to people as opposed to the other way around. I'm only half-joking when I say that I'd like to put people on the bridge of the Starship *Enterprise*. Everyone would have a simple setup. There would be a screen and all you'd have to do is talk to your computer, let's call it Harry. You'd just have to ask Harry for anything you need and it would automatically get done. You know, 'Harry, call my doctor.' 'Harry, it's an emergency, dial 911.' 'Harry, get me a Lyft or an Uber.' 'Harry, which one of my friends nearby is home right now?' It has to be that simple."

And soon, it may be. Lenovo Health, a health IT company based in Triangle Park, North Carolina, and Orbita, a Boston-based company that develops connected home healthcare, have teamed up to create Lenovo's Smart Assistant, a voice-controlled speaker for the home that embeds Amazon's Alexa voice platform in Harman Kardon speaker technology. And this is just the beginning of turning virtual assistants—voice-activated robots—into our personal healthcare managers. So one day in the near future, it may really be possible to say, "Alexa (or Google Home, or whoever) take my blood pressure, reorder my medication and have that drone deliver it right to my door."

This is an example of the new wave of interface design—techies call it "Zero UI," meaning no user interface. Although talking to a computer is not new, the combination of speech recognition, cloud computing and machine learning allows for a level of interactivity that can approximate interactions with a person for simple conversations and tasks. As I will discuss in Chapter 5, this will be refined in due time to allow the computer not to just recognize the words, but also the emotional content underneath them. We'll look back on typing at a computer keyboard with the same fondness we now have for rotary dial telephones!

It stands to reason, if someone is overwhelmed or not feeling well, or is not tech savvy, introducing new technologies that require any effort may be asking too much. The inability to solve this problem could be the major impediment to adoption of connected health. In later chapters, I'll be talking about companies that have taken on this challenge and created very simple technologies that fall into the plug-and-play category. But, there is still a long way to go.

Culture Shift

More than anything else, the culture of healthcare needs to change before there will be system-wide changes. The new value-based versus volume-based reimbursement models encourage teamwork, a true shift for doctors who have been pretty much trained to be loners. Under conventional fee-for-service models, doctors are the rainmakers, their reputations bring in the patients who pay the bills. The staff is typically deferential to the doctors, as are many patients. Cost containment is not a high priority. Doctors are unlikely to call each other out over unnecessary testing or other inefficiencies that pad a bill. And the patients who pose the greatest economic drag on the system—the ones who end up in the emergency department or require long hospital stays—are the cash cows for providers.

Under newer models that focus on value and outcomes, it's no longer "each doctor for himself." It's about the team—and that includes the patient. In a connected health model, doctors are no longer the "seers" who have all the magic tools; patients would have access to the same tools to gather their own data. There is a shift in responsibility, and perhaps doctors recognize that when they cede some control to patients, they are no longer put on a pedestal.

It might take a whole new generation of physicians, who have been trained differently, to fully embrace the connected health model of healthcare that I outlined at the beginning of this chapter. And that's exactly what California-based Kaiser Permanente has in mind for its innovative medical school, which is scheduled to open in 2019. Kaiser is a nonprofit insurance plan that runs its own hospitals and clinics; its physicians are paid a salary. And that makes a big difference in how they do business. Kaiser is already ahead of the curve in terms of connected health. More than half of its interactions with patients are through telehealth, a sign of what's to come when value-based models supersede fee-for-service.

Christine Cassel, MD, planning dean for Kaiser's new medical school, is the former CEO of the National Quality Forum and was a member of President Obama's elite President's Council of Advisors on Science and Technology (PCAST). Cassel says that Kaiser Permanente's medical school will be the first medical school housed within a high-functioning healthcare system, rather than a university or research center. "Kaiser is taking a very different approach to medical school education," she explains. "The concept is to immerse the student in a healthcare system that works. We don't just want to give students a class about teamwork or about systems; we want them to actually see it in action every day and have the real-life experience be part of the lesson."

Cassel notes that patients will be helping to design the curriculum. "We have Kaiser members and patients on our curriculum commit-tee and our faculty council. We've embedded the voice of the patient throughout the school, in terms of the governance and in terms of the curriculum, to help all of us, including the doctors and educators, re-member that very often we see it from a different perspective than the patients."

According to Cassel, connected health will be baked into the medi-cal school curriculum, part of the students' everyday interactions with patients. "We're in discussions with several of the big technology com-panies right now about partnering around the technology infrastructure for the school," she says. "And the medical students will eat this up. It comes very naturally to them."

Cassel adds that this isn't just about changing the culture for doctors; it's also about changing the culture for patients. She notes that if the move to value-based reimbursement models continues, by necessity it becomes imperative that patients become more engaged and take more responsibility for their health. "Patients have to start thinking of the healthcare system as a partner to keep them healthy, not as the place you go only when you don't feel well," she explains.

Although there are patients who already are active in maintaining their wellness, it's not the norm, according to Cassel. "Unfortunately, lots of chronically ill people still take a relatively passive perspective on their care, but I think that's going to change."

But how soon will any of this happen?

If I had to guess, my hunch is that the Kaiser Permanente School of Medicine will be very successful because it will be integrated into a healthcare system that puts the patient first, uses a multitude of modern tools to engage with them and does not carry the classic tension between providers and payers that leads to balkanization and lack of cooperation. It could provide the model that eventually cracks the chicken or the egg conundrum, or at least overcomes some of the hurdles that have been keeping the healthcare system locked in the past.

◆ ◆ ◆

INTEROPERABILITY: WILL IT HAPPEN IN OUR LIFETIME?

The healthcare system will soon be overwhelmed by an influx of older patients, many with complicated conditions, taking multiple medications, being treated by numerous healthcare providers. Many of these patients may have cognitive problems that make it difficult for them to keep track of their ailments. And even the sharpest of individuals could easily forget to report a previous procedure or medication when they are filling out the intake questionnaire in the doctor's office.

Will there ever be a time when a patient can walk into any clinic, hospital or specialist's office, anywhere—and *voilà*—the medical staff will have access to that person's complete health record? The free exchange of healthcare information, regardless of origin, would be great.

Having said that, I have to add a caveat: In my time in healthcare, I've never seen interoperability achieved. It appears that the one thing business models for medical technology suppliers, health plans and providers have in common is that they all value high switching costs for their users. Even in cases where interoperability allegedly exists, it is not robust. One example is Digital Imaging and Communications in Medicine (DICOM), the standard for radiologic images. Various vendors can claim to be DICOM compatible, but still their systems don't talk to each other.

Health plans want to keep members on their rolls and providers have little interest in making it easy for patients to receive care at a competitor. We already know tech companies view information sharing as a vulnerability. Interoperability requires tremendous investment on the part of current market participants and, since no one has a business model that welcomes interoperability, it never goes anywhere. For example, the Continua Design Guidelines have been available for over 10 years and are acknowledged as an international standard for personal health systems. Recently, the Design Guidelines added remote monitoring for diabetes care, hypertension, heart failure and chronic obstructive pulmonary disease, but have been slow to gain real traction.

For some reason, standards-setting bodies in healthcare IT have not achieved what other industries have. Although not exactly comparable, think how easy USB, Wi-Fi and Bluetooth have made our lives. For health tech, perhaps it has to do with the fact that the end users of the service (patients) don't pay the bills. They can't vote with their wallet in any meaningful way to support an interoperable model.

But I am not convinced that interoperability is the biggest barrier to moving the market forward, though it is a favorite topic for technologists and policy wonks. I agree it would be nice to have, no question. But do we need really it to move the market forward? Maybe not. There are a number of favorite barriers to telemedicine adoption—interstate licensure being one example. They are all important, but I've chosen to devote time and energy to problems that are solvable.

When and if there is a time that interoperability will be essential for moving the market forward, it will happen quickly, according to Robert Havasy, MS, senior director, HIS, HIMSS North America. "We don't have interoperability today because the market doesn't demand it. And as soon as we get the business drivers correctly aligned, and information sharing provides value to healthcare organizations, we'll have stunning interoperability in a matter of months. There are almost no technical problems with interoperability. They're all related to a lack of will, which is caused by market forces."

At the moment, the will doesn't exist. To make it happen, we need one of two things to occur (or ideally both). Government policy levers could be pulled. This might be done by only reimbursing for care from providers using an interoperable system, giving tax breaks to companies that are interoperable, only purchasing interoperable software for government purposes and other similar strategies. Secondly, if there were some rising-tide-floats-all-boats scenario, where all of the EHR companies could benefit by interoperability, it would start to happen. There are examples of this in other industries. Why did VHS vs. Beta become a war, whereas Wi-Fi and USB became standards?

Simply put, until there is a business model for interoperability, challenges will remain in seamlessly collecting and transmitting health data between personal connected health devices, providers and caregivers.

CHAPTER 4

From Reactive to Proactive: Taking the First Steps

"Almost everything in healthcare is done after someone is having symptoms or is already sick or has fallen off the wagon. We need to move beyond chasing disease toward more predictive models. We need to be alerted when something negative is happening that may not have an immediate impact, but could become a problem within the next 30 to 60 days. And we need to know the right interventions to avoid that problem. This will save money by preventing a hospital readmission or visit to the emergency department, but it may also encourage patients to pay more attention to what's going on with their own bodies. Perhaps, one day, people will get to the point where they can figure out how to solve some of these problems for themselves."

—KAMAL JETHWANI, MD, MPH, SENIOR
DIRECTOR, CONNECTED HEALTH INNOVATION,
PARTNERS CONNECTED HEALTH

"To me, it comes down to individuals owning their own health behaviors and health decision-making process. Do I just assume that I hand my care over to the professional? Or am I provided the opportunity to learn what's actually happening to my body and how my personal decisions and actions will impact that? Am I taking personal responsibility for my health and healthcare? A big part of making this happen is providing the right educational resources to consumers."
—SARAH THOMAS, SENIOR DIRECTOR OF
GLOBAL INNOVATION, GENESIS REHAB SERVICES/
GENESIS HEALTHCARE; EXECUTIVE-IN-RESIDENCE
AND INNOVATION FELLOW, AGING 2.0

Healthcare in the twentieth century was focused on caring for the sick. It was—and to a large degree still is—stuck in a *reactive* mode. We tend to wait until there is a problem before we intervene. I'm not only talking about the healthcare *system*, I'm also talking about healthcare *consumers*. Ours is not a prevention-oriented culture where consumers are expected to do their part to stay well. If that was the case, I doubt we would be burdened by the current epidemic of chronic disease that is aggravated—if not initiated—by lifestyle. Just look at today's older adult population, where chronic disease accounts for some 86% of total healthcare costs. And then there's the personal cost, in terms of robbing people of their health and vitality in their later years. If the healthcare system were proactive, if people were trained from an early age to step up to the plate and manage their health, we wouldn't be seeing such a gap between healthspan and lifespan.

When people complain that the healthcare system isn't focused on prevention, I agree with that assessment, and I know that we can do more. But the reality is, there's only so much we can do from the top down to keep people well. I suspect that this will hold true for as long as we have a healthcare system. Active management of one's health is the key concept here and, arguably, this concept has increasing importance the older we get. We also have to keep remembering the basic economics of healthcare: There will be too few healthcare professionals to care for too many sick people. There will be too few young people to pick up the tab for the growing numbers of ill elderly. The only way to reduce this burden is to empower and encourage people to do more for themselves, not only in terms of self-care when they do fall ill, but in terms of prevention. And that requires a real paradigm shift in how healthcare is delivered.

I know that selling preventive health is tough, especially to the young. Early in life, the body has a resilience that nicely matches the "I am indestructible" youthful mindset. Nature's feedback loops can compensate for lifestyle neglect or excess. As time goes on, the natural cellular and organic aging processes lead to a physiologic state that is less tolerant of environmental or lifestyle changes. The failing heart can't tolerate even the slightest change in dietary sodium. Likewise, bad kidneys require careful attention to fluid and electrolyte balance. Type II diabetes requires diligent carbohydrate monitoring. Complicating matters is that, in many of these examples, there is little if any symptomatic warning of impending health deterioration.

Connected health tools have provided us with a number of new capabilities, including the means to measure and track aspects of our health that we may otherwise have been unaware of (steps, activity, weight, blood pressure, etc.). There is a strong case to be made that this type of tracking (and the resulting feedback loops) is a critical strategy at both an individual and population level if we are to move beyond a reactive "sick-care" system to a proactive healthcare system. This, in turn, will have a direct effect on longevity. This chapter is about that challenge.

I understand that there will always be people who, due to genetics, bad luck or other life difficulties may fall ill. We will never have a population that is 100% healthy. But we can do a lot better to improve the healthy score than we're doing right now.

I don't mean to paint a completely negative picture—we've done a really good job in some areas. The longer lifespan we now enjoy is widely acknowledged to be due, in part, to a decline in deaths from heart disease, thanks to aggressive cholesterol screening and treatment with statin drugs, though the data shows that adherence to these drugs is alarmingly poor (think about how much better off we'd be if we could improve it!). Vigorous public health campaigns against smoking have also significantly reduced the percentage of Americans who smoke cigarettes and the anti-smoking message can be tied to longer lifespan. The knowledge we've gained over the past century about the inner workings of the human body has enabled us to develop drugs and other therapies that can extend life.

I'm very pleased to report that there is another encouraging development on this front. Tens of millions of Americans have taken the initiative to use a wearable device to track fitness levels, daily activity, blood pressure and/or heart rate. They are using digital health devices and health apps like iHealth and Nokia (formerly Withings), smart scales and MyFitnessPal, and wearing Fitbits, Apple smartwatches and the like. This is a good sign: It is the beginning of people becoming proactive in a grassroots way and we need to nurture this phenomenon.

Now, I recognize that half of all people who use digital devices to track their health stop using them within a few months. That may be true, but I prefer to take the "glass half-full" approach: The fact that half keep tracking their health suggests that about half of us are intrinsically motivated by these feedback loops. This is a great start, but we need to figure out how to motivate the other half of people who quit midstream. And more importantly, how do we attract the majority of people—including the aging population—who may be skeptical of digital health, put off by what they perceive as difficult technology or worried that they will fail.

We still haven't done well enough in promoting healthy behavior changes that could significantly reduce, if not reverse, the chronic disease epidemic. It's not for lack of trying. The problem is multifaceted and solving it will require multiple strategies.

Although most doctors regularly encourage patients to eat better, get more exercise, reduce stress and the like, they only have 20 minutes or less with each patient during an office visit. That's barely enough time to deal with the purpose of the visit, let alone gain a deep enough understanding of a patient's behavior patterns or habits to know how to motivate them to make healthier lifestyle choices. And the fact that physicians don't get reimbursed for lifestyle coaching, as I noted earlier, is another chicken or egg issue that is clearly blocking progress on this front. To compound the problem, most doctors are not really trained in preventive health. Most of the clinical training we receive in medical school and residency is about dealing with acute illness. New reimbursement models that reward efficiency, lower-cost and team-based care provide us with a roadmap to move in the right direction.

A second challenge is that the effects of lifestyle choices today do not accrue, usually for years or even decades. I have a legion of patients who say to me, "If I only knew when I was younger what sun exposure would do to my skin." The human brain is wired to focus on near-term events and discount long-term consequences. This well-known behavioral economic principle is called delay discounting (or time discounting), which means that the longer it takes to reach a goal, the more willing we are to take a smaller or immediate reward as opposed to waiting for a bigger long-term payoff.

Health is a *very* long-term payoff—and there are many temptations along the way that derail us. At times, we all succumb to the "I'm eating this donut because it will make me feel good *right now*" urge. The fact that not eating it will keep me healthy and vigorous in my old age just isn't that important at that moment. These days 70% of healthcare costs are lifestyle-related and thus impacting these costs will require us to learn how to bypass this powerful instinct. We haven't done it yet.

Related is the ambivalence people feel about being accountable for their health outcomes. The very notion of health insurance implies that random bad luck events will happen and that we should have a mechanism to pay for these. That puts us in a passive, reactive mindset. It flies in the face of current knowledge of disease prevention. In addition, we are by nature a libertarian society. We have the right to engage in unhealthy behaviors and we've made (wittingly or not) a societal pact that says we'll bear the cost of those indiscretions.

Lastly, the value of prevention is ephemeral. Let's go back to the smoking example I provided above. Lowering the rate of tobacco consumption has clearly been linked to health benefits. Watch a few episodes of *Mad Men* and you'll see how far we've come. But can we say that the effect of reduced tobacco consumption has been lower cost of care? That is a much harder argument to make. The government is overwhelmed with paying for sickness (the Medicare trust fund is headed for bankruptcy). Employers and health plans tend not to find return on investment (ROI) in prevention because people move from job to job and plan to plan. It can be years before they can harness the downstream benefits of a plan enacted today.

The promise of connected health is that it will overcome these hurdles. It will be a highly personalized approach to preventive medicine designed to accommodate the needs of each individual. Backed by a deeper understanding of the interplay between genetics, disease progression and human behavior, this new "holistic" approach would enable us to anticipate and even nip many potential problems in the bud. It will help people stay healthy and vital for as long as possible.

To oversimplify the strategic approach, we need to:

- create incentives for doctors to engage in prevention and provide the appropriate training. We have made some progress with this on new payment models;
- change our cultural view of healthcare from one where everything is bad luck or an accident to one where some accountability is both accepted and encouraged;
- combine the push toward value-based reimbursements with investments in public health prevention.

The Vision

What role can connected health play in this? I'm not presumptuous enough to suggest that I have all the answers, but for the past 20 years at Partners Connected Health we've been laying the foundation for a new way of practicing medicine. Everything we do is focused on giving people the tools they need to participate in their healthcare and to make the system more responsive to the immediate needs of individuals. From our inception, we had a vision of a smarter, personalized, patient-centric, efficient system that could deliver care anywhere, anytime. We are moving in that direction. And here are some of my thoughts about where we are headed.

I understand that once people have become set in their ways, it's hard to get them to change, so the earlier we start, the better. If we want to extend the healthspan, we need to begin early. Under ideal conditions, true proactive healthcare would begin at birth. Based on the genetic profile, each newborn would be assigned a highly personalized healthcare program to guide him or her through life, to minimize the chance for illness. This program would learn over time from phenotypic and environmental inputs. It would be a comprehensive approach—the ultimate in what we now call complementary medicine—combining medical intervention with lifestyle. Each plan would include targeted strategies on optimal diet, exercise, sleep and stress reduction specific to each person's unique genetics, physiology and psychological profile.

Proactive healthcare would extend beyond the annual physical exam or occasional screening test or procedure. It would move out of the medical office to become a continuous, fluid interaction with individuals conducted in real-life settings. All patients—or at least those at higher risk—would have the option of using connected health tools to gather personal health data in real time. These tools would be effortless, discreetly incorporated into the objects that we use every day, creating what we at Partners Connected Health have dubbed, the "Internet of *Healthy* Things."

As my colleague Kamal Jethwani mentioned above, predictive science could take much of the guesswork out of the practice of medicine. Sophisticated predictive models could identify subtle changes in either biometrics or behavior that could portend future problems. Armed with this information, we could quickly intervene to ward off health issues or lessen their impact.

If someone does get sick, the treatment could also be highly personalized, based on the patient's genetics and other data. And individuals would be able to manage their medication and other therapies in a much more proactive way, consulting in real time with virtual coaches, who could intervene as often as needed.

Early in life, parents would implement proactive healthcare on the behalf of their children, until they were old enough to assume the responsibility themselves. It's not unrealistic to think that some of this information would be used to guide women through their pregnancies—or even help them to get pregnant—to optimize the health of their newborns. A big part of this vision is the constant input of individual data from wearables and mobile devices. This data forms a unique digital fingerprint that can be used as a measurement tool/feedback loop/moment-by-moment reporting system. The data can also be used as fuel for the analytics that will drive the highly personalized, engaging health improvement program that will accompany each of us from "cradle to grave."

At the moment, the vision of a truly proactive healthcare system is more imagination than reality. It may take another generation before we achieve the goal of hyperpersonalized "lifetime wellness" to significantly reduce today's burgeoning chronic disease burden.

For starters, we won't get there unless there are substantial changes in how healthcare is funded. That's a given. I'm going to make the assumption that some of the chicken or egg issues discussed in Chapter 3, like payment models that favor in-person, face-to-face interactions, eventually will be solved simply because they will have to be.

Second, individuals will be asked—even required—to step up to the plate and manage their healthcare in a way that they were never expected to in the past. It will necessitate a massive retraining of health consumers, empowering them with simple and intuitive technology and providing them with targeted and timely incentives to keep going.

Third, we can't afford to wait for decades to change how we deliver healthcare. I attend numerous health conferences and meetings each year, and there is a tendency on the part of visionaries to gloss over the present and move rapidly to a discussion of the ideal. Contemplating the model scenario for healthcare is useful in terms of helping us understand the steps we need to take to get there. But the aging population and the increased burden this places on the system make it imperative for us to find ways to deliver high-quality healthcare in a more effective, efficient and economical manner, *right now.*

And most importantly, we need better ways of engaging patients so that they feel both empowered and responsible for managing their healthcare as they partner with physicians and other healthcare providers.

The Age of Specialization

Given all the challenges facing the healthcare system—including an aging population, too few healthcare personnel, sicker people and the skyrocketing costs of drugs—you might think that all concerned would be eager to try something new. But a shift from reactive to proactive health is not simply a matter of automating medical records or creating programs for people to share personal health data with providers from their homes. A proactive system is a true paradigm shift that is a radical departure from how healthcare has been practiced for several generations.

This fundamental change in healthcare delivery will take cooperation on the part of providers, payers and, most importantly, consumers. The bottom line is: If we can't get people to embrace this new way of doing health, it won't work.

More than a half-century ago, the creation of Medicare ushered in the era of medical specialization that resulted in a change in the economics of healthcare and (predictably in retrospect) the behavior of doctors. It also helped promote the reactive "treat the problem" approach that is still ingrained in the healthcare system today. As noted previously, the government "gift" of insurance for the elderly and infirm led to increased demand for services. As individual services were paid for, volume of service delivery increased.

When I was in medical school in the early 1980s, we were taught the "primacy of systems." We didn't look at the "whole patient," but were instead taught to think of patients as collections of organs that could be damaged by diseases. For example, we would look at kidney disease as an electrolyte/acid-based condition. Similarly, we were taught to view heart disease as an arterial blood flow challenge, not a problem caused by a sedentary lifestyle, excess stress or poor diet. Many of us came to think of our patients as physiologic laboratory specimens. You have high blood pressure? That is a physiologic process gone wrong. This sounds harsh and is not intended to fault my colleagues who virtually all assume they are doing the very best for their patients. It is really pointing out the culture we were trained in—it was all about fixing organ systems gone wrong.

At the same time, our growing knowledge of how the human body works gave rise to the modern pharmaceutical industry. As a result, we could offer patients more effective drugs, but perhaps, in the process, we minimized the importance of lifestyle. Many patients may have also thought, "Gee, if this medication can keep my blood pressure normal, why should I bother exercising or eating healthy?" As it turned out, drugs alone didn't keep disease at bay. And of course they have side effects and, often, downstream unintended consequences.

What snuck up on us was the change from a disease burden primarily of acute illness (e.g., infectious diseases) to a disease burden of chronic illness, which most experts agree is up to 70% lifestyle related. When you looked at it that way, the physiologic specimen approach I described seems very narrow-minded. It's just been within the last few years that we've seen meaningful changes in how doctors view illness. But we've only recently begun to change our care models and processes to include team-based care, as well as lifestyle coaching, mind-body influences, mindfulness and the like. Value-based reimbursement has helped and will continue to do so. These factors are encouraging team-based care, but the pendulum is swinging slowly.

Consumers: Still on the Fence

From the consumer perspective, the new model of proactive healthcare is also a radical departure from how healthcare is delivered today. Under the present system, the bar has been set pretty low. All we expect from patients is that they (1) show up for their appointments, (2) take their medication properly and (3) alert us when they have a health problem. As long as someone else pays the bill, or the cost of care is nominal, most patients appear to be content with the status quo. If we are to truly transform the healthcare system, we need to give people the tools that provide them with continuous and meaningful support as they go about living their lives.

When it comes to using persuasive technologies to encourage behavior change, we often talk in terms of carrots and sticks. Certainly, creating tools that engage and motivate is important, but part of this process is to convince people that they need to use them in the first place. Yes, sometimes we need to go back to square one!

But not everyone is ready or willing to take responsibility for health. The premise of proactive healthcare is that an optimal lifestyle, and prompt intervention if things go awry, will keep you well. In other words, individuals have a great of power over their own health. This seems so basic to those of us in healthcare that we may forget it is not so obvious to the general public.

There are still a large percentage of people who don't see—or who don't want to acknowledge—the connection between their actions and health outcomes. In fact, according to the 2016 Ipsos International

Survey on Connected Health, the *majority* of the people they polled in the United States fail to see the connection:

- Only 44% of people polled agree with the statement, "I am in control of my health."
- Only 40% agree, "The main thing which affects my health is what I actually do."
- Only 38% agree that, "If I get sick, it is my own behavior which determines how soon I get well."

If, as this survey suggests, most people don't even recognize how their behaviors impact their health, we are failing to deliver health information in a way that is resonating with them. Based on his interactions with patients, Kamal Jethwani is not surprised. As he points out, "A lot of people don't think of their illnesses as preventable and their health events as avoidable. I don't think people make the connection between lifestyle and habits or understand that the input and output mechanism—what you put in your mouth, what you eat or drink—can actually impact your health. People don't make that straight-line connection between, if I eat X today it's going to affect me in this way tomorrow or 10 years from now."

Data as a Teaching Tool

Connected health can help "connect the dots" to enable people to better understand how their behavior impacts their health. A case in point is Partners HealthCare at Home's monitoring program for patients with congestive heart failure who have been recently discharged from the hospital or are at risk for rehospitalization. Each morning, patients take their blood pressure, pulse, oxygen levels and weight using wireless monitoring devices that capture their personal data. In addition, patients answer symptom questions on a small touch-screen computer and transmit all of this data to Partners HealthCare at Home, where a telemonitoring nurse reviews the data. If the readings are outside established parameters, appropriate intervention is taken. Since we launched the program in 2003, we have seen a significant decrease in readmissions and visits to the emergency department, which reduces the burden on the system.

What has made the program so successful is that it's not just about gathering data; it's about educating patients so that the data becomes meaningful—and actionable. Daily monitoring, structured education and "just in time" teaching from our staff on topics like nutrition, medication adherence and exercise help make the connection between the numbers and patients' actions. Patients have told us, "I had no idea that eating a can of soup for dinner, which contains a lot of salt, could cause such a big weight gain the next morning," or "On days that I talk a walk, my numbers are better." Patients surveyed said that the program increased their confidence and improved their understanding of heart failure and how to better manage their condition, as well as helped them avoid rehospitalizations.

Here's something that I found really interesting: Although there is less face-to-face interaction with these patients, they report feeling more connected and better cared for with our home monitoring program. The reason is that they have *constant* connectivity. In one of the patient's own words, "My nurse calls me *before* I get short of breath."

The beauty of CHF home monitoring—and similar programs— is the authenticity. We get the opportunity to understand how people conduct themselves in real life and use this information to correct behaviors and intervene as necessary to improve health outcomes.

Someday, it may be possible to identify people at risk for CHF decades earlier to correct the problem, before their heart muscle gives out and treatment becomes a challenge. But right now this type of real-time intervention is making a real difference in the lives of these patients.

A Window into Real Life

I noted earlier that, given the typical rushed interaction during an office visit, even the most well-meaning doctor can't learn enough about a patient to design a program that will not only resonate at the moment, but become incorporated into that person's life. Patient-generated data provides a window into an individual's habits and lifestyle, particularly about the person's technological engagement level and ability to achieve personalized tracking goals.

Humans apply filters and biases when they estimate about themselves. I'm no different. When my doctor asks me each year how much I exercise, I always reply, "Twice a week." What I neglect to add is " . . . *on a good week.* " I'm not trying to deceive him, but that's just how the answer always comes out.

I don't mention that during weeks when I'm traveling, or have some other commitments, I may only exercise once a week or not at all. If my doctor had access to my actual activity data, and if it was trended and analyzed for him, he'd be able to say, "Actually, you exercise an average of 1.3 times per week and since we're shooting for 3 times per week, let's put a plan in place to get there." And, of course, I'll be able to follow that plan very carefully because my connected tracking device is linked to my calendar. By understanding my habits as well as my real-life obligations, my doctor—and eventually my virtual health coach—can offer more precise advice to keep me on track and healthy.

Advances in artificial intelligence could get us to the point where much of this intervention and advice is automated. I look forward to the day when Siri or Alexa will know my schedule, and say, "Joe, I see that you're going to be staying at a hotel in Washington, D.C., which has a great gym. Why don't we schedule a 40-minute workout session for you next Tuesday? And you can do your other two workouts after work on Monday and Friday."

One important key to success is to find the right engagement tool to make a lifestyle change stick. Devices that capture patient data serve as a source of truth that can enable a richer teaching experience, and not just for sick patients. These can be tools to promote wellness.

Tough Love

Recently, the "my health isn't my responsibility" way of thinking is starting to change, in large part because consumers are now being forced to foot more and more of their own healthcare costs. The "consumerization" of healthcare, triggered by rising premiums, copays and drug prices, is making people aware of health costs in ways they never were before. According to *U.S. News & World Report*, experts estimated that for 2016 alone, "The share patients will pay for their care will increase. Out-of-pocket costs this year will hit $350.1 billion, and are expected to rise to $555.8 billion during the next decade. Part of this is occurring because employers are increasingly shifting medical costs to employees, often through high deductible plans."

This financial impact may provide some motivation for consumers to reduce costs by staying well or encourage them to shop around for the best plan. The reality is, many people don't really have a choice: Either they must use their employers' plan or buy whatever is available in their market.

But not just consumers are motivated to reduce costs. Employers and insurers are offering incentives to keep people more engaged in healthy activities. Even big box pharmacies like CVS and Walgreens are luring consumers with innovative ways to stay healthy and earn rewards in exchange for engaging in healthy activities like participating in weight loss or smoking cessation programs or wearing an activity tracker.

This realization sparks both debate about privacy and consternation about being held accountable for health targets—and punishment for missing them. "Will my employer fire me for not walking enough?" "Will my insurer charge me more?" "This all sounds very creepy." These are some oft-repeated refrains.

Health-tech devices allow us to measure engagement and outcomes. Thus, if you equip people with these tools, you can either reward or punish them for certain behaviors. There are a couple of examples of successful rewards programs: Walgreens Balance Rewards; the UnitedHealthcare Community Rewards and HumanaVitality Rewards.

Two interesting posters presented at the 28th Academy of Managed Care Pharmacy Annual meeting in April 2016 in San Francisco caught my eye. The first showed that people who tracked their activity four or more times a week were "associated with significantly higher adherence and optimal adherence to antihypertensive and antihyperlipidemic medications" for Balance Rewards members 50-plus. The second reported that Balance Rewards members who used the Walgreens mobile app pill reminder feature had significantly higher adherence to oral antidiabetic, antihypertensive and antihyperlipidemic medications. I understand that the participants in these studies were motivated enough to join Balance Rewards and use a tracker or app, but nevertheless, I think it demonstrates what can be accomplished if we get people on board.

UnitedHealthcare also offers a Community Rewards program that enables members to accrue points for healthy behaviors, like preventive doctor visits, getting immunizations and completing their health assessment quiz. Members are asked to track these and other healthy behaviors they engage in every day (like being active, brushing their teeth and making smart food choices) online. Each activity earns points, which can be cashed in for gifts in the online rewards catalogue. (This is a separate program from its Motion program mentioned earlier.)

Another program, HumanaVitality Rewards, uses incentives and rewards to promote behavior change, doling out Vitality Points and Vitality Bucks for activities such as taking your health assessment, logging daily steps with a tracker or getting preventive screenings. In 2016, Humana reported on a three-year study of 8,000 employees on its HumanaVitality Rewards program. Based on that study, participating employees "had fewer unscheduled absences, lower overall health claims costs and fewer visits to the hospital and emergency room."

As noted above, the right incentives seem to work without resorting to arm twisting. Yet, there's also been a great deal of discussion about using more coercive tactics to promote better health habits. In other words, if someone wanted to smoke, eat junk food or skip a medication, that person would have to pay a great deal more for healthcare than someone who was more health aware or compliant.

Will we ever implement this type of punishment for poor health habits? Will we actually reward people for eating carrots and passing on the cheesy bread sticks? I am skeptical. It is really not the American way to punish someone for lack of health-related accountability. Look at the uproar over the Affordable Care Act's individual mandate, requiring all residents to maintain health insurance that meets minimum coverage standards—or else you could be taxed. If citizens are unwilling to simply take responsibility and purchase their own health insurance, it doesn't bode well for taking this to the next level, giving individuals responsibility for their own health. And let's face it; based on results from the Ipsos study, it's clear that we still have a long way to go to convince people that they are an important part of their own healthcare.

However, it may be possible to achieve the same impact without using such a big stick. For example, an insurer can offer a lower premium cost to members achieving certain health-related outcomes, as measured by engagement with apps or data from devices. That same insurer can also raise the "standard premium price" over time, so that those who don't achieve these health goals are, in effect, being penalized. I don't think it will ever be advertised as such, but noncompliant members will feel the pinch in their wallets.

Making Health Addictive

Somehow we have to recast health tech from being a tool that reminds us that we're sick or threatens us with a future illness if we don't do as we are told. We have to move beyond scolding people for not meeting their goals, denying them items of pleasure and making health look like a distasteful chore. This is especially challenging because so much of chronic illness is lifestyle-related and requires the trade-off between short-term pleasure and long-term gain. We need to do this artfully.

In my last book, I devoted a chapter, "Try a Little Dopamine," to ways we can make health addictive. Since writing that book, I've developed a bit more understanding of what makes software (on mobile devices, anyway) addictive. Beyond what I already covered in the previous book, I now realize that we must use software to establish trust and empathy. In addition, we must respond emotionally and, of course, harness motivation, which often includes a social experience, such as game mechanics. Folks are trying this, but it is in its infancy.

The odd thing is, the best way to engage people in their health may be to not talk about health—or disease—at all. At Partners Connected Health, we realized early on that simply spitting data back to people wasn't going to get them engaged. So we spent a great deal of time thinking about the best ways to encourage people to become proactive in their health.

A few years ago, we came up with the concept of "making health addictive." By "addictive" we meant finding ways to make interaction with health tech as compelling as other experiences that keep us coming back for more, like our smartphones. Since the introduction of smartphones, I have been fascinated by their addictive qualities. With no prompting, the average person looks at his phone about 50 times a day. Some people never put them down. I have written about how smartphones trigger the same feel-good "dopamine" response in the brain as other addictive activities. I have also urged health-tech developers to try to elicit those same qualities in their tech-to-human interactions.

Based on our research and experience with patients, my team and I came up with three strategies and three tactics for engaging people, which we try to incorporate into the design of new health technology.

The three strategies for engagement are:

1. *Make it about life.* Don't focus on disease, especially for wellness apps.
2. *Make it personal.* Sound like you are talking to the user, not to every other person using the app or device.
3. *Reinforce social connections.* Enable people to share their experiences within their social network.

The three tactics are:

1. *Employ subliminal messaging.* Unobtrusively insert messages promoting healthy activities when people least expect it.
2. *Use unpredictable rewards.* Offer random presents, discounts and the like to encourage usage.
3. *Use the sentinel effect.* Let users know that someone is watching and evaluating what they're doing.

In the time since we first wrote about "addictive health," our team has been inspired to add a new strategy, one that may be the most important: *Design interventions with empathy.* We have learned that it's critical to create a bond between the user and the technology, a feeling that "it" really understands you. And, most importantly, that "it" understands what you're going through.

System designers have long known that if software can be trained to empathize with users, it more quickly establishes a bond and "tricks" the brain into humanizing the software program. This can be done by incorporating mundane features like emojis and push notifications that seem relevant to what is going on in the user's life. There are also more sophisticated "emotion enabling" technologies on the horizon, such as software that can decode facial expressions and analyze emotions in real time, as well as voice analytics that can do the same thing working with speech patterns. (More on this in Chapter 5.)

We will keep getting better and better at this, to the point where we will be able to match the right interaction to an individual's precise mood and needs.

The future state will be software that knows you well enough to know what the best way is to motivate you. For example, some people may require handholding, more sympathy and understanding; others may respond better to a drill sergeant coaching style.

At times, empathy may be exactly what a patient needs and, oddly enough, a digital device may be able to do as good a job, if not a better one, at making patients feel cared for than a human being.

Put yourself in the shoes of a cancer patient taking strong painkillers to manage her pain and suffering from a typical side effect of those drugs, a severe GI problem, in this case constipation. She needs to know if there's anything she can do to alleviate her problem, or if there's anything else she can do to feel better in general. This was the patient we had in mind when our team designed ePAL, a mobile phone app created for patients who are taking strong painkillers to control their cancer pain. The original purpose of ePAL was to make it simple for patients to contact their oncology service by phone when they had a problem or a question, but it included other features that patients seemed to "bond" with.

We conducted a pilot program with the Palliative Care Center at Massachusetts General Hospital, in which one group of patients received the ePAL app and one group did not. Every morning, patients with the app were asked to rate their pain and then were given specific advice about how to adjust their dose based on that rating. The app was an at-your-side companion that gave the patients a set of in-the-moment answers to questions related to cancer pain control. The app checked back in two hours to see if the patient felt better. It also provided information on how to deal with common side effects of opiates, like GI problems. The app also offered a comprehensive library where patients could learn about alternative ways to manage pain, as well as get information on optimal diet, exercise and stress management techniques.

Despite the fact that it was easier than ever to contact the oncology service, the rate of phone calls actually went down among the app users. At the same time, patient pain scores improved significantly compared to the control group (a 40% improvement), as did their self-reported quality of life.

My colleague Kamal Jethwani attributes the success of the app to the fact that patients did indeed form a bond with it, as we had hoped—perhaps even a stronger bond than they could form with a human provider.

As Jethwani explains, "A lot of our patients were completely surprised that someone even bothered to ask them about their pain every day. That's a question no one asks them, and no one really listens when they talk about it. This is an interface they can be pretty honest with, without feeling judged. It cares about things that they care about, that no one else is really caring about and no one else has the time to talk to them about in the same way. They can take their time finding an answer and they can read through information as many times as they need to before finally understanding. They don't have to worry about wasting someone's time or appearing uninformed. They know that a computer doesn't judge them. And perhaps people bond with the app so strongly because they feel they're not being judged."

At Partners, we are also exploring the potential to use data in ways that can improve our ability to apply predictive analytics. Our goal is to understand not only when a patient will require intervention—which of course is important—but even more so to determine which type of intervention will work best for each patient.

Toward that end, we are using data collected from smartphone usage and social media interactions to build algorithms that determine who is a good candidate for which type of intervention. As Jethwani further explains, "For example, we are collecting data on how many times you post on Facebook or Instagram, how many times you comment, how many times you tweet or re-tweet. We're looking at what kind of content you're both viewing and engaging in, and whether that is negative or positive. Then that tells us a lot about people and their motivations."

To follow up on that, if someone uses social media mainly as a tool to observe other people, and doesn't interact, offering them an intervention that requires a great deal of social interaction is probably a mistake. "How you use social media tells us a lot about you as person and we can start to integrate that intelligence into our interventions," Jethwani says. "What does your smartphone utilization tell us about you? What you do with your free time tells a lot about what you like to do and what might motivate you. Then we can start building that intelligence into healthcare interventions, because we want to make them fun and engaging, especially if we're talking about prevention."

Most of all, we need to make our interaction with health tech feel personal and show that it understands and cares about us as individuals. Advances in AI are fast making this a reality. Your smartphone, tracker, laptop and personal assistant will soon be able to "read" your emotions, in real time, and respond to your needs. And this will make our digital devices an even more indispensable part of our lives.

◆ ◆ ◆

PRIVACY: SOME THINGS TO CONSIDER

We talk a great deal about what we can learn about patient data, and how it can improve healthcare, but we need to remember one thing: As long as there is connected health and patient data, the issue of privacy will keep cropping up. I've thought a great deal about this and have come to the conclusion that there is only one answer. People need to feel that they are getting some value back for giving away their health data. In other words, they need to feel that whatever risk they may be incurring is worthwhile.

When it comes to data and privacy, people seem to focus on two possible threats. First, that their insurers or their employers will use their data against them. Second, that their personal data will be hacked and fall into the wrong hands. What I find interesting is that, for the most part, people seemed to have made their peace with the potential risk of data breaches as a result of using credit cards. In years past, hundreds—if not thousands—of companies from Neiman Marcus to Yahoo, Zappos and Target—have been hacked. Certainly, there have been many more commercial data breaches than hacks of medical records. But despite the ongoing and persistent threat of data breaches, we don't see people cutting up their credit cards, deleting their social media accounts, skipping shopping online or avoiding hotel stays.

We all know how much more secure chip readers are for our credit cards and how easy it is for swiped machines to get hacked. Has that stopped people from using swipes when no chip reader is available? Not in my experience. The convenience of using credit cards is too great.

The reality is, people understand that there is risk whenever they socialize online, or send an email or text—yet they keep doing it. Once again, that's because they perceive that the value of communicating in a virtual setting exceeds the risk. We need to do a better job of explaining the benefits that can be accrued from the sharing of healthcare data. Patients need to be informed of what they stand to gain by having an accurate, up-to-date electronic health record or of how their personal data may one day be used to predict an illness that could be prevented with earlier intervention.

And maybe we need to address some of the nightmare scenarios that keep people up at night. It may be difficult to prevent all data breaches, but we can prevent some of their negative impact. For example, people are concerned that insurance companies will use their data to exclude them from coverage, raise their rates or, even worse, share their personal health data with their employers.

There are some policy levers in place that should help with this. The Affordable Care Act has a clause that makes it illegal for an insurer to deny coverage. At this writing that law is still in force, but I have seen it do little to quell the fears of data misuse. HIPAA makes it illegal for insurers to share data with employers, yet the fear persists.

Fear of hacking is rational. We have to make the value proposition for data sharing so strong it becomes as widely accepted as the use of credit cards.

CHAPTER 5

Reading People

"If we can understand you better through your data, we can nail down what motivates you. We can then use that to get you to live a healthier lifestyle. People don't care about their healthcare for healthcare's sake. We need to find the key to what you do care about."
—Kamal Jethwani, MD, MPH, senior director, Connected Health Innovation, Partners Connected Health

So far in this book I've talked a great deal about the gap between the lifespan and the healthspan, and the difficulty we face in getting people to take steps to maintain their own health. Artificial intelligence tools that not only track behavior, but correlate behavior with specific physiological and emotional changes, could give people a better understanding of how their thoughts and actions impact their health. And the simpler these tools are to use—the more they blend in with people's everyday lives—the more likely people will be to use them.

What can be simpler than talking? Imagine the following scenario: You get a text from your doctor asking you to book an appointment and you agree to a televisit for later that day. During your virtual meeting, your doctor reassures you that everything is fine . . . for now. But based on ongoing analysis of your voice patterns, the system projects that you are at high risk of developing coronary artery disease within the next two years. So, your doctor reaches out to discuss some preventive measures to keep you healthy. And then she asks, "Maybe you haven't been feeling quite like yourself lately? The software also noticed a slight change in your speech that suggests that you may be getting a bit depressed."

The idea that disease could be detected in its earliest stages by monitoring your speech may sound a bit farfetched, but scientists, investors and even the US Army are taking it quite seriously. There is a growing body of scientific research linking subtle variations in speech patterns over time to the onset of emotional or physical ailments. These speech variations are called vocal biomarkers. The human ear can't detect them in their earliest stages, when it would be most valuable to identify a problem, but the right software can.

Why all the interest in voice? For most of us, it seems effortless, but the act of speaking is one of the most complex physical actions that anyone can undertake. Speaking involves hundreds of active muscle fibers working in tight coordination and multiple circuits in the brain that cover a significant percentage of brain activity—including hearing what was said in a dialog with others, processing it and deciding what to say in response.

"All this activity involves three major systems—the central nervous system, the muscular system and the respiratory system," explains Jim Harper, PhD, co-founder and chief operating officer of Boston-based Sonde Health. Jim is also entrepreneur-in-residence for PureTech Health (also in Boston), which invests in early stage technologies and where he is a member of the venture creation team. "What we're seeing—and what investors are looking at carefully—is that with the right contextual data, you can train these AI models to recognize objective changes in voice that reflect changing physiology in these three major systems that are occurring across a range of diseases." Jim came to me early on when Sonde was an idea and a bit of technology. It's been exciting to watch the company take shape. Interacting with Jim has given me a new appreciation for the power of voice analytics.

Founded in 2015, Sonde Health is a self-described "digital medicine company," developing a voice-based technology platform with the goal of transforming the way we monitor and diagnose mental and physical health. What makes voice analytics particularly interesting is the ease in which data can be collected, in real time and in real life, via objects people use every day: smartphones, tablets, home robotic assistants and the like. It could provide a simple way to remotely monitor a large number of people to detect diseases like high blood pressure, Type 2 diabetes and coronary artery disease in their very earliest stages, before the damage sets in and when they are easier to treat through lifestyle changes. For those of you who may be thinking that this sounds a bit too intrusive, understand that these tools analyze the *quality* of your voice, not the content. They are not meant to eavesdrop on private conversations, but merely to detect and track changes in vocal patterns.

Every time you ask Siri a question, or talk to Amazon's Alexa, Google Home or Microsoft's Cortana, you are providing voice samples. From the perspective of consumers, it's easy and unobtrusive (as long as it's done with your consent!). From the perspective of researchers, your voice data could provide a treasure trove of information about you. The tricky part is analyzing that data, finding common distinguishing factors in people's vocal patterns that can be correlated to a medical problem and then creating the algorithms to track those factors—vocal biomarkers—in a large population.

Voice analytics is part of a bigger trend to tap the technology that we use every day to provide a deeper look into human life. This new field is called emotion AI. It includes a broad spectrum of technologies that can capture and infer human emotion from voice, language, facial expressions, gestures, body posture and physiology, and any combination thereof. With every virtual interaction—when we text, speak, shop or take a selfie—we leave behind a digital fingerprint. Mining that data could provide heretofore hidden insights into health and wellness as we age. It could also provide a means of detecting subtle physiological changes that would normally go undetected, but could be a sign of a developing problem. This is the proactive medicine of the future.

Voice analytics isn't new. Voice analytic software to track emotion has been used for some time in call centers around the country ("This call may be recorded for quality and training purposes.") For example, insurance companies, banks and sales agents use this technology to identify callers who, depending on the circumstance, may be angry or upset and need special handling. What is new with voice analytics is its focus on health and wellness, and the growing recognition that we need new tools to combat chronic disease.

Your emotional response to different situations could provide important clues about which types of health strategies might work best for you. One of the most frustrating parts of practicing medicine is that we pretty much know ways to reduce the risk of disease, but our patients don't always heed our advice. As a dermatologist, I recommend that people slather on the sunscreen when they're outdoors, but many don't listen until they show the first signs of skin cancer.

Today's trackers give us mostly quantitative information (steps, hours of sleep, blood pressure, weight, etc.). To integrate this information into healthcare in a way that truly brings care as a continuous function into your life, we need the emotional context. The kinds of technologies featured in this chapter provide both emotional context for our tracking numbers (i.e., were you inactive yesterday because you were depressed or because it was rainy out?) and another avenue for tracking through the mind-body connection. The latter may be even more impactful to our future. The role of these technologies in longevity mustn't be missed. As we get older, it is harder to move around and get out of the house. With a full suite of biomarker assessments, we'll be able to focus on those individuals who need help and bring it to their doorsteps proactively.

Voice isn't the only innovative disease biomarker on the horizon: Other companies, like Boston-based Affectiva and San Diego-based Emotient (which was acquired by Apple in 2016), are looking at facial decoding—analyzing facial expressions—as a means to track and measure emotional states. This technology is also being explored as a tool to detect depression, suicidal tendencies and other cognitive problems.

These tools may not only be useful for diagnosing potential health problems, but can provide an objective measure for gauging how well a medication or other therapy is working. And this data is not just for providers or payers. If put in a meaningful context, it could be very useful for consumers who want to gain insights about their own behaviors.

Finding Your Voice

Speech is becoming a rich source of information about health and many companies and research centers are working on a wide range of projects in this area. For example, a Parkinson's disease iPhone app called mPower, developed by Seattle's Sage Bionetworks and the University of Rochester Medical Center, gathers real-time data from Parkinson's patients, including voice samples, to better understand the disease. Parkinson's patients often have low speaking voices and may slur their words. The app, which has been used by about 15,000 patients as of this writing, can measure the severity of disease by analyzing subtle changes in voice.

Another startup, Cogito, is an MIT spin-off co-founded in 2007 by Joshua Feast and Alex "Sandy" Pentland, PhD, head of the

Human Dynamics research group at the MIT Media Lab. Cogito received funding from the Defense Advanced Research Projects Agency (DARPA) and other investors to "develop an artificial intelligence platform and behavioral models to interpret human communication and detect psychological states automatically." The company's voice analytic technology has been used by the US Department of Veterans Affairs to help veterans with post-traumatic stress disorder (PTSD), as well as improve call centers for healthcare organizations and commercial enterprises.

If you thought that the heart disease scenario presented at the beginning of this chapter was a bit too "out there," think again. Tel Aviv–based company Beyond Verbal conducted a preliminary study with the Mayo Clinic to see if they could find a "distinguishing factor" in voice that could detect early heart disease. They presented their findings in a poster session at the American Heart Association Scientific Sessions in November 2016 ("The Sound of Atherosclerosis: Voice Signal Characteristics are Independently Associated with Coronary Artery Disease"). Using a smartphone app developed by Beyond Verbal, Mayo researchers studied 121 patients who were scheduled to have coronary angiography, as well as 25 control patients. "All subjects had their voice signal recorded using an application downloaded to their personal smartphone device prior to the coronary angiography. Voice was recorded, stored and analyzed for multiple features of voice intensity and frequency using 'Beyond Verbal Communications' clinical trial application." The researchers concluded, "We identified abnormal voice characteristics that are independently associated with CAD. This study suggests a potential relationship between voice characteristics and CAD."

Beyond Verbal is currently conducting a study in China to see if the results can be replicated in Mandarin.

Sometime in the future, it really may be possible to diagnose a heart condition or neurological problem by analyzing a phone conversation. At the moment, most medical testing is not quite that simple.

Conventional biomarker development has focused on identifying molecular biomarkers, whether from blood, saliva or another sample taken from a patient. Analysis is done at a laboratory and the process is inherently costly, as well as inconvenient for patients, especially older people with mobility issues. This poses a barrier that could discourage many from doing it at all. In contrast, voice biomarkers would be effortless on the part of patients, and samples could be easily obtained through the very tools people use in their everyday lives—phones, tablets and virtual assistants.

Sonde's Jim Harper predicts that "passive" data collection is going to be one of the key disruptors of medical testing and that voice, "the richest data source in the space," will lead the way. Sonde has licensed voice analytic technology developed by MIT's Lincoln Laboratory. The lab invented technology that identified biomarkers in a person's voice to detect signs of mental health problems, including depression, mild traumatic brain injury and Parkinson's disease. In October 2016, Lincoln Lab partnered with the US Army Medical Materiel Agency (USAMMA) to create algorithms that can detect mild traumatic brain injury, or a concussion, based on vocal biomarkers.

Harper says that although mental health is an important subcategory, Sonde has a much broader mission. "We are looking beyond the indications that have been published to date and exploring a number of possible areas where vocal biomarkers are likely to exist. Validating that changes in voice can be objectively measured for a range of conditions in cued speech gives us additional confidence that allows us to prioritize the best targets moving forward, where we can have the greatest impact," he explains. "It's an approach of quick discovery and validation based on the platform that we are building around voice analytics, while engineering the passive capability in parallel, so that when it's available we'll be able to roll out products very quickly."

Training and validation of vocal biomarkers typically begins by obtaining a range of brief voice samples from volunteers with and without a particular condition. These samples are used to identify multiple subtle acoustic changes that correlate with a disease or symptom of interest. Machine-learning models are then built that combine these correlated features to maximize overall accuracy for assessment outputs that objectively measure the presence and severity of the particular disease or symptom. For example, the volunteers may be asked to read or repeat a syllable or phrase to capture specific articulations, describe the weather or a hobby to get free speech examples or perform verbal tasks designed to elicit or evaluate specific cognitive, emotional or physical states.

The samples would then be compared/analyzed for identifiable vocal biomarkers—in other words, identifying what acoustic changes are shared in common by individuals with a symptom or condition that are absent in individuals without it. From this research, you can create the algorithms to (1) identify existing medical conditions and (2) eventually be able to predict potential problems that may crop up down the road.

Harper groups potential biomarkers into three categories:

1. *Persistent vocal biomarkers.* These reflect transitions to atypical or diseased states that are chronic and persistent—they can last for weeks, months or even years. Persistent vocal biomarkers should enable strong correlations with more traditional disease diagnoses for the likely presence of conditions like dementia, major

depressive disorder, Parkinson's disease, chronic obstructive pulmonary disease and heart failure.

2. *Dynamic vocal biomarkers.* These vary on much shorter time scales and reflect more transient neurological or physiological states or symptoms. They would be similar in practice to vocal features correlated with mood or affect, which can change rapidly based on environmental stimuli. But these vocal features correlate with objectively measurable and clinically meaningful states like respiration rate, heart rate, blood pressure, muscle coordination/tremor, cognitive load, stress, sleepiness, etc.

3. *Hypothesized predictive vocal biomarkers.* These may be persistent or dynamic vocal biomarkers, but instead of being selected and trained to correlate to a state present at a given moment for diagnostic or monitoring purposes, they are trained *retrospectively.* That is, they use longitudinal data to look for specific features that reliably *precede* a particular change in state or symptom (e.g., a response to a therapy, onset of a disease, acute exacerbation or relapse, and so on). There is insufficient data at present to determine how reliable or widespread these biomarkers may be and how far in advance they may provide actionable information. Sonde's goal is to build new data at scale to allow this hypothesis to be tested.

If this research pans out, Harper says, it would provide proof that changes in the voice are an objective measure—that is, provide a vocal biomarker—for specific conditions. Eventually, it would prove the authenticity of predictive vocal biomarkers. And that could really make a difference for the early diagnosis of disease.

For some conditions, like depression or other cognitive disorders, there are no objective medical tests for diagnosis. In the case of depression, clinicians must rely on patient self-reporting or their own observations during the brief interaction they have with their patients. While some patients may be very insightful and capable of expressing their emotional state, others may mask their true feelings or be unaware of them or their significance. As a result, depression is often misdiagnosed, goes undiagnosed or takes a long time to be diagnosed.

There are several companies, including Sonde, racing to invent voice software that can run unobtrusively in the background but alert health professionals if a patient is experiencing depression or even suicidal thoughts. Of course, any form of passive tracking would have to be done carefully, with the consent of the consumer and all the appropriate privacy protections.

Alzheimer's disease is another condition that is very difficult to diagnose in its earliest stages. Harper notes that there have been numerous drug trials for Alzheimer's treatments, but none have panned out. One of the factors accounting for these failures could be that these trials target patients in the later stages of the disease, when their brains are already overtaken with amyloid plaques, and most of the damage has already been done. Furthermore, the cost of finding patients with bona fide Alzheimer's disease versus cognitive impairment is very expensive and inefficient. "Right now, finding patients for these studies relies on PET imaging at a cost of $10,000 or more per patient. Even when the initial screens are done, the number of patients that are amyloid positive can be as low as 20%," he explains.

Harper is hopeful that voice analytics could provide a solution for these and other difficult to diagnose problems. "That's why we're so interested in good clinical data, which has been missing from a lot of voice correlation studies to date. The better we can correlate vocal biomarkers to burdensome and costly clinically validated measures of disease, the more power and accuracy these models will ultimately have," he says.

Written All Over Your Face

Vocal analytics is one way to gain insight into the physical and emotional state of human beings, but there is an even more obvious source of data—the human face. Less than 10% of communication is conveyed through the content of the message, our words alone. We discern the true meaning of words from nonverbal cues like body language and tone of voice—but especially from reading each other's faces. For most human beings, the ability to decode facial expressions is hard-wired in our DNA.

Understanding and responding appropriately to the emotions of others is the hallmark of emotional intelligence, or emotional quotient (EQ). More than IQ, EQ is considered to be the number one predictor of success in all aspects of life. In fact, we know that people who have severe problems with EQ are often unable to make key decisions in their lives, keep jobs or build relationships. On the flip side, people with high EQ are more likeable and persuasive, and have more successful careers and personal lives.

Computers traditionally have been built for high IQ; they are loaded with cognitive skills, but lack EQ. Now that we are spending more and more of our lives in the virtual space, there is a growing movement among technologists to build computers with EQ—that is, giving computers the ability to discern human emotion. There are several startups on the cutting edge of the emotion AI space, which, as I noted earlier, is the science of training computers to read and respond to human emotion.

Rana el Kaliouby, PhD, a pioneer in emotion AI, is co-founder and CEO of Affectiva, a company that she spun out of the MIT Media Lab in 2009. She is a star both in terms of her scientific contributions as well as her entrepreneurial spirit. El Kaliouby predicts that in the near future, our smartphones will be embedded with "emotion chips" that track our emotional state, just like they currently have GPS. And just like you can share your activity tracking or purchasing information with friends, you will soon be able to share your emotion data with whoever you want. And all of these inputs from steps to voice to facial recognition are synergistic when they are combined in a machine-learning environment.

El Kaliouby and her team created Affdex, software that enables computers to detect and analyze human emotion in real time. Using a basic webcam found on any computer, tablet or smartphone, Affdex reads facial expressions and matches them to corresponding emotions. It can reveal what people feel in the moment (e.g., happy, sad, disgusted, engaged or confused). It can rate how intensely they're experiencing the emotion and track fluctuations in emotional state, second-by-second, in real time. This technology can read facial expressions across genders, cultures and age ranges.

Affectiva's software has been used by Fortune 500 companies as a market research tool, but el Kaliouby feels that there is also an enormous potential in healthcare. Affectiva has worked with the autistic community, creating software to help autistic children and young adults better interpret emotional cues. The company is also working with a suicide prevention specialist to create a tool that enables therapists to identify people who are at highest risk for suicide, so that they can intervene before it's too late. You can see the parallels with the voice analytics companies and their aspirations.

El Kaliouby notes that in the past it was enough for computers to have cognitive smarts, but now, in their new role interacting with humans, they need to have emotional savvy. "This is especially true for an AI system that will need to interact, communicate and coexist with humans, which is increasingly true for AI systems," she says. "For example, a social robot or virtual nurse caring for an older person needs to have cognitive AI—it needs to know how to dose the medication. But without emotional AI as well, these systems will be unable to truly understand their users, build a strong rapport with them or be effective in bringing about behavior change."

The example of medication adherence is a perfect one. Depending on the ailment, patient outlook and insurance coverage, nonadherence rates can range between 25% and 50%. Experts estimate that poor adherence can cost the healthcare system around $300 billion annually in hospital and doctor visits due to complications that arise from not taking medicine as directed. And as more and more specialty drugs, like biologics, are coming on the market with price tags that can reach the high five figures, there's great interest on the part of providers, payers and drug companies to make sure that these medications don't go to waste. We know that forgetfulness is a minor component of adherence. In fact, a recent paper demonstrated that, in general, smart pill bottles and reminder systems were not effective in improving overall adherence. Imagine if "the system" not only knew you might be forgetting and when, but also your concerns and fears about side effects, your ability to pay for the medication and the financial tradeoffs you are making, to cite just a few examples. If we wrap in Affectiva's facial recognition smarts with voice analytics and a smart pill bottle, we could make a real difference.

El Kaliouby adds that the nonhuman advisor or social robot will need to be able to identify if someone is in pain, unhappy or even lonely, so that it can try to improve the situation. For example, a social robot needs to know when to contact a friend, relative or medical personnel to intervene.

How do you teach a hunk of metal and plastic to understand emotion? Affdex is grounded in the international Facial Action Coding System (FACS), a taxonomy of facial muscle movements developed by Swedish anatomist Carl-Herman Hjortsjö and refined by American psychologist Paul Ekman and others. In emotion science, each facial muscle movement is called an action unit. According to FACS, there are 46 basic facial actions—spontaneous and subconscious shifts in facial expressions, like the raise of an eyebrow, the curl of a lip or the furrow of a brow. Each one may last for only a millisecond, but they are accurate indicators of a person's precise mood. For example, action unit #12 is a lip corner pull (or pull of the zygomaticus muscle), which is the main component of a smile. Action unit #4 is the brow furrow (or pull of the corrugator muscle), the drawing together of the eyebrows that is a strong indicator of a negative emotion. Teaching a computer to read facial emotions is hard; the 46 facial action units can be fast, subtle and combined in a thousand different ways to portray hundreds of nuanced emotion states.

Twenty times each second, Affdex samples about 20 facial expressions, or "emotion data points," simultaneously. The software then analyzes them for expressions of seven basic emotions—happiness, sadness, surprise, fear, anger, disgust and contempt—as well as for more complex emotions such as interest and confusion. Affdex puts the raw data in context, weaving a highly personalized narrative about each subject. (Unlike facial recognition programs used by law enforcement, Affdex does not link to a central database to correlate faces with names.)

Even the most highly sophisticated computing programs can't duplicate the precise and elegant method by which humans process information, but they are getting tantalizingly close. Affdex uses a methodology called deep learning, a highly sophisticated form of AI, to create a face-reading algorithm (software). In deep learning, computers are taught to solve a problem or identify an object or emotion by building on its experiences, just like humans do. The goal is to endow the algorithm with the ability to continually upgrade itself, then tweak and fine-tune its knowledge base as it accumulates more data.

Emotion recognition tools are incredibly exciting to me and the future is bright. However, two big hurdles must be overcome to see this go into widespread use. First is the fact that cameras are now only on our devices. So to do emotion recognition we must be interacting with a device. Second, of course, is the "creepiness factor" and respecting people's privacy. One can't underestimate that—however this is done—people need to feel as if they aren't being spied on or imposed upon.

El Kaliouby herself acknowledges this. She takes a strong position that there needs to be value—such as a better experience with your device, personalized content or better connections with people you care about—in return for sharing data as personal as your emotions. In other words, as I've state earlier, there has to be something in it for the user that makes the loss of privacy worthwhile.

Feelings Are What Makes Us Human

The same software that teaches humans how to "read" people better can teach machines to do the same. That's why emotion AI is needed now more than ever. As our digital devices become embedded in our lives, it will be essential for them to act more like humans and less like machines. When you're asking a conversational agent a question about your medical condition or medication, the last thing you want (or need) is a response that is brittle, feels dismissive or appears uncaring. You wouldn't be happy with that behavior from a human being! If we are to move people to health tech, the tech itself must be humanlike enough so that we feel some connection.

More and more, it's becoming second nature to turn to technologies like Siri, Cortana and Alexa when we have a problem, even a serious, personal crisis. In May 2016, *JAMA Internal Medicine* published a study that tested the ability of four widely used smartphone assistants—Apple's Siri, Microsoft's Cortana, Google Now and Samsung's S Voice—to adequately respond to questions regarding mental health issues, rape or domestic violence. They pretty much flunked. At the time, Siri didn't even recognize the phrase "I've been raped" and none of the assistants understood "I am being abused" or "I was beaten up by my husband." Only Siri knew enough to refer someone to an emergency medical service upon hearing the words *heart attack.*

The study's researchers, from University of California, San Francisco, and Stanford University, concluded, "When asked simple questions about mental health, interpersonal violence, and physical health, Siri, Google Now, Cortana and S Voice responded inconsistently and incompletely. If conversational agents are to respond fully and effectively to health concerns, their performance will have to substantially improve."

The study quickly trended on Twitter and Facebook, attracting a great deal of attention from the media. It made headlines like "'Siri, I Was Raped': The Woefully Inadequate Way Smartphones Respond in Crises," and "Hey Siri, Can I Rely on You in a Crisis? Not Always, a Study Finds."

It's easy with 20/20 hindsight to ask, "How could the 'geniuses' that designed these virtual agents not have anticipated this would happen?"

Keep in mind, all of this is very new and probably took them by surprise. The more people used Siri and other conversational agents, the more comfortable they felt with them, and the more they wanted to reveal about themselves. Suddenly, Siri was put in the role of confidant and therapist, which it was never intended to be.

There is a lesson to be learned from this study. As we begin to rely more on health tech, like digital coaches, to implement behavior change for example, our virtual helpers need to know the best way to interact with us at any given moment. If you're experiencing a personal crisis and are turning to a social robot for help, at the very least it should be able to get you assistance. In some cases, it really could be a matter of life or death. If you're using a digital tool to stay fit or lose weight, it should know when you may need prodding, or handholding, or when it may be best to leave you alone. It may mean the difference between you actually sticking to a wellness plan or turning off the device and putting it in a drawer. As noted above, the next phase of health-related sensors will include multiple inputs that allow us to gauge your emotional state. This is critical to realizing the vision of time-and-place-independent care and to caring for citizens as they get older.

At Partners Connected Health, we are always looking deeper, trying to figure out why people behave the way they do, so we can provide the best intervention. If we understood the emotional context behind biometric readings like blood pressure or glucose levels, or how a person felt the moment he decided not to go to an exercise class or skipped his medication, we could better frame solutions that might work better for each individual.

When it comes down to it, the power of AI in healthcare is not to spy on people or collect as much data as possible. The real strength of AI is its ability to provide information that can help forge stronger relationships between individuals and their healthcare providers. If done correctly, AI–enabled tools will help solve some very difficult problems in healthcare by reaching out to people in a way that conventional tools can't.

Introducing the home robot—and it's not much bigger than a breadbox.

For the past two decades, MIT Media Lab alum Cory Kidd, PhD, founder and CEO of San Francisco–based Catalia Health, has been working on how to apply robotics to patient engagement and healthy behavior change. When he was at MIT, Kidd partnered with Boston Medical Center to create a diet robot that helped overweight patients lose weight. An early trial done at the center showed that people responded so well to the diet robot, they not only lost more weight than a control group, but they didn't want to part with the robot at the end of the study. In 2008, Kidd launched his first company, Hong Kong–based Intuitive Automata, which offered Autom, a diet robot for the home. Autom was just a bit ahead of its time. Although the work at Boston Medical Center proved that it was an effective weight loss tool, the technology was very expensive and difficult to scale.

Kidd knew that his company had been on the right track in terms of using robotics as an effective tool for engagement, but he was left with several questions, including, "Where is there a customer who's willing to pay for it?" The answers to that and other questions were what really led Partners Connected Health to work on applying this technology around chronic disease management and medication adherence.

In 2014, Kidd launched Catalia Health and its robot Mabu, a personal healthcare companion that uses AI to "create a real relationship" with the patient. Mabu is short for *mabutaki*, a Japanese word meaning "to blink" and *mabudachi*, or "best friend." Designed by IDEO, an international design and consulting firm headquartered in Palo Alto,

California, Mabu is about the size of a small kitchen appliance, with a camera embedded within its body. It has an appealing face with big eyes that can make eye contact with the user. It is holding a touch screen. Mabu is an "expert" in psychology and is "emotion enabled" with Affdex software that allows it to track human faces and decode facial expressions. Mabu can move her head up and down, and speaks in a pleasant, soothing female voice. Unlike most apps that offer medication adherence services, like daily reminders, Mabu doesn't sound like a broken record—she engages users in a different discussion every day, targeting their personalities and moods. The average interaction is two to three minutes.

As I write this, Catalia's clients are major pharmaceutical companies that are offering Mabu free to patients to help improve medication adherence and provide advice on how to implement healthy lifestyle changes. Many users are older patients who are managing multiple health problems—some are late-stage cancer patients—and are on complicated and expensive drug regimens.

Mabu is designed to be remarkably easy to use. Patients are notified by their provider or pharmacist that they have been selected to be offered Mabu. The robot arrives in a box and all the patient has to do is plug it in and Mabu begins the conversation. As Mabu learns more about the user, the conversation becomes more personal. Based on earlier studies, Kidd says that patients working with Mabu showed a 40% improvement in engagement, which meant that they adhered to their medication regimens 40% longer than controls.

I am thrilled to hear about this straightforward approach to distribution and set up. For years at Partners Connected Health, we have observed that simple is critical. As I mentioned in Chapter 2, the phrase in the industry now is "Zero user interface" (Alexa and Siri are examples of Zero UI). We need to continue to make these technologies easy to set up and use if we are going to realize the vision of connected health for longevity.

Although Kidd's early work had been in diabetes management and weight loss, he notes that there are many similarities between those fields and medication adherence. "When I was in the clinic at Boston Medical Center, I worked alongside doctors, dietitians, nutritionists. Our typical patient had tried and failed at several diets over the past two years. The whole reason that they came to us was that they wanted to succeed," he explains. "They believed that they were really going to do it this time. We have that motivation intrinsically—most people want to get better. Most patients actually want to succeed on treatment. A lot of what we're trying to do through Mabu is help people to achieve their own goals. We want to give people a tool to help them stick with something that they already want to do." The concept there was if we can make healthcare goals about near-term life goals, we should do much better in achieving self-motivated health improvement.

Despite Mabu's high-tech bells and whistles, Kidd says it's not about technology, but rather about the relationship—and that requires a deep knowledge of psychology. Kidd explains, "It comes down to how do you create, build up and maintain a relationship over time? We know that many people don't take their meds properly, but it doesn't make much sense to talk in general terms to someone about taking their medication. The reasons people aren't taking their meds vary from patient to patient. It depends on whether we're talking about a patient with a late-stage cancer, or someone with a chronic disease that they've been dealing for decades, or a young person who's just been diagnosed and has been told that he's going to have to take a drug for the rest of his life. We need to understand the challenges for that particular patient population."

Mabu has been "taught" to carry on a discussion with a user that can adapt to the user's particular needs. "It's really about taking psychological theories of relationship and using that to create the AI algorithms that are going to develop conversations with each patient," Kidd says. "The patient doesn't hear the same thing every day; we actually try to tailor the conversation based on everything we know about that individual. Are you the kind of person who just likes to be told what to do and you're going to go do it? Do you want more explanation about why you're going to do this? In a way, we're trying to read the person, the way people try to read each other. We are asking questions, getting a response, understanding what that means in terms of the psychology of this individual and how we should best approach him. We're trying different things and we're seeing which ones work."

Of all the trends in technology, the move to intuitive, responsive interfaces that "read people" may be the most important, especially in light of the aging of the world's population. Much of today's technology (e.g., smartphones, wearables, and the like) requires a level of manual dexterity, mental acuity and sharp vision that can discourage their use among older people who may be experiencing some physical or even cognitive decline. I suspect that this may be one reason why older adults (70-plus) have been avoiding smartphones. They may be put off by the small screen and tiny keyboards.

Voice-activated interfaces like Alexa, Siri and Cortana, although not yet perfect, are a major step forward. But in order for our technology to be truly "seamless," it needs to blend into our lives to the point that we no longer have to think about it. It's there when we need it—for example, it can alert us (or our loved ones) if we are in danger or heading for trouble.

As we have seen, technology that understands vocal or facial cues may even be able to detect health problems long before there are obvious symptoms. But the beauty of this technology is that it disappears when we don't need it—it doesn't feel like an added burden or something else to learn or do. To paraphrase the nurse who expressed his concerns in Chapter 3: It needs to be effortless.

CHAPTER 6

Managing Chronic Disease

"I'm a primary care doc and in a typical practice you see the patient for maybe seven or so minutes. The best you can do is tell them, 'Eat less, exercise more, take your medicine. Good luck. I'll see you in three months.' They come back in three months; they haven't done what you told them to do. You say, 'You bad noncompliant patient.' The cycle continues. This is hard. If it were easy, we wouldn't have this problem. What we're paying for right now is what doctors do—which is diagnoses and treatment. That is very different than executing on 'the plan.' That's the part that we don't do well in US healthcare."
—RUSHIKA FERNANDOPULLE, MD, MPP, CO-FOUNDER AND CEO, IORA HEALTH

When it comes to acute care, for the most part our healthcare system excels in serving the needs of patients. When it comes to managing the chronic disease epidemic, however, it is falling short. As Rushika Fernandopulle, who's quoted above, observes, the healthcare system is not designed to help patients sustain the kind of behavior changes required for chronic disease management.

We are paying dearly for this deficiency. The older adult population is especially hard hit by chronic diseases like Type 2 diabetes, lung disease, coronary artery disease, arthritis and cognitive impairment (which may be triggered or aggravated by a chronic disease). According to the National Council on Aging (NCOA), about 80% of older adults have at least one chronic disease and 68% have at least two. Chronic disease accounts for 86% of total healthcare costs in the United States. These are "stealth diseases," so-called because they are often symptomless until they have caused significant damage to the body. If untreated, or poorly managed, they can result in serious complications down the road and a diminished quality of life.

Why are we losing the chronic disease battle? I addressed this issue in a commentary published in *Nature Biotechnology* in March 2016, which I co-authored. I wrote then, "Simply put, the bulk of chronic disease development and management occurs beyond the reach of the healthcare system. Patients need intervention before developing disease, and those with chronic disease need ongoing and consistent support from multiple layers of providers to bring about behavior change."

The inability to provide these services goes back to the chicken or the egg dilemma. As I noted in the *Nature Biotech* piece, reimbursement for preventive care has been "spotty." As a result, the burden of managing chronic disease pretty much falls onto the patient.

Managing one or more chronic diseases after they occur can be very difficult and time consuming. People often have to take multiple drugs throughout the day, stick to a special diet, try to get enough exercise and, on top of all of that, have to track blood sugar, blood pressure and/or their weight. This can be overwhelming for someone at any age, but it can be especially challenging for the frail elderly or those who have some degree of cognitive impairment. If you've got great insurance or lots of money, you can hire people to ease the load, but that's not the case for most Americans. Caregiving falls to family members, who are often torn between their jobs, their own children and the needs of an older relative. They do the best they can, but most can't provide care in real time.

There is growing interest in creating a new paradigm for the prevention, treatment and management of chronic disease, using new tools made possible by the Internet of *Healthy* Things. We now have wearable trackers, mobile computing platforms and social media that can help keep patients informed and engaged in real life, real time. These new technologies will be paid for by stakeholders who are drowning in rising healthcare costs, including employers, consumers who are faced with rising premiums and copays, public and private payers, and healthcare systems switching to value-based reimbursement plans. The big challenge is migrating there from our current pay-for-sick system. Those who pay are wary of short-term increases in costs as we begin to reward healthy behaviors while still having a significant burden of sickness to pay for. There is hope as more and more providers enter risk-sharing arrangements with private payers and Medicare moves forward aggressively with its pay-for-value agenda. What is lagging, however, are the care models to facilitate ideal performance under these new payment models. It will be critical to accelerate adoption of the care models that work if we are ever to surmount the challenge that comes with the growing number of older adults and their healthcare needs.

This chapter features three examples of companies employing creative approaches in this area:

- *Omada Health.* This company delivers a digital curriculum based in part on the NIH's groundbreaking National Diabetes Prevention Program.
- *Iora Health.* Iora is offering a "whole new operating system for healthcare" that focuses on the needs of Medicare patients.

- *Care.coach*. This platform provides "care and companionship" for seniors in the form an interactive virtual health coach.

While these are three great examples, there are many more innovative companies tackling this chronic illness management problem. I chose these in particular because I have been an advocate and student of the founders of each of them as they have built out their businesses. I've watched Omada's ascendency with great interest; I know Rushika, the CEO of Iora, through his Massachusetts General Hospital connections; and I have been on the advisory board of care.coach and its predecessor, GeriJoy.

The New Epidemic

I'm not suggesting that everyone can be a "superager," programmed to stay vital and healthy well into their late decades. Along with lifestyle, luck and genetics also play a role. But our genetics haven't changed over the past century and I doubt that as a population we've run out of luck either. Yet, we have seen a rapid rise in many chronic diseases and one in particular—diabetes.

When we talk about the diabetes epidemic, we're talking about Type 2 diabetes, a condition characterized by the inability of the body to use insulin properly. Type 1 diabetes, which typically strikes early in life, is an autoimmune disease in which the body does not produce enough insulin. In contrast, Type 2 diabetes is associated with obesity, a sedentary lifestyle and poor diet; it is more common among people in midlife and older. When I was in medical school, Type 2 diabetes was called "adult-onset" diabetes, but in the 1990s the name was officially changed to "Type 2" because, for the first time, it was being diagnosed in children. This oddity was attributed to the rise in obesity among children, another modern phenomenon that can't be blamed on just genetics and bad luck.

A highly publicized study led by Edward Gregg, PhD, chief of the Epidemiology and Statistics Branch, Division of Diabetes Translation, National Center for Chronic Disease Prevention and Health Promotion in Atlanta, included diabetes incidence in the United States from 1985 to 2011. Gregg's team found that the lifetime risk of developing diabetes had doubled for an average 20-year-old American man, from 20% to 40%, during that time. The rate of increase for women during that time was 27% to 39%.

Based on statistics from the American Diabetes Association (ADA), more than 25% of Americans over 60 years of age have diabetes. Every year, 400,000 Americans 65 and older are diagnosed with diabetes, primarily Type 2 diabetes. If untreated or improperly managed, diabetes can lead to stroke, heart attack, blindness, neuropathy, limb amputation, kidney failure and premature death. It's not only a very serious condition, but diabetes is also very expensive. According to the ADA, prediabetes and diabetes cost the US economy about $322 billion a year. The ADA notes that healthcare costs for someone with diabetes are about 2.3 times what they would be for someone without this disease.

You don't become diabetic overnight—it is often preceded by a "prediabetic" period. According to the CDC, 86 million Americans over the age of 20 have prediabetes, a condition characterized by higher than normal blood sugar levels, or elevated HbA1C in the range of 5.7% to 6.4% (6.5% is bona fide diabetes). Studies show that if caught early enough, Type 2 diabetes can be prevented and even reversed. This requires a significant change in lifestyle, notably weight loss and careful diet management, as well as exercise. As anyone who has ever broken a

New Year's resolution to lose weight and get to the gym knows, this type of behavior change is very hard to sustain on your own.

There are several startups tackling diabetes prevention, but Omada Health, which I profiled in my earlier book, *The Internet of Healthy Things*, has conducted multiple clinical studies with older adults. It's worth taking a second look at this innovative company. Omada is known for its streamlined, easy-to-use technology, which isn't surprising considering the two co-founders, Sean Duffy and Adrian James, met at IDEO, the San Francisco–based design firm. Duffy was doing an internship as part of an MD/MBA program at Harvard. James headed the Medical Products domain for IDEO's Health and Wellness Practice. They struck up a friendship and decided to create a "digital behavioral medicine company" to ease the burden for people living with chronic disease. Their first ambitious goal: Turn back the diabetes epidemic by nipping the problem in the bud, before the disease could take hold.

In 2011, Duffy and James launched Omada Health, a company that delivers a digital version of the face-to-face NIH National Diabetes Prevention Program. Omada Health's program is a year-long online, interactive behavior change program that mixes technology with real-life coaching. In March 2015, it was one of three digital programs to achieve pending recognition from the CDC as meeting the Centers' evidence-based standards of the National DDP. The program is available to participants via any laptop, tablet or smartphone. Named one of the top 10 innovative companies in health for 2017 by *Fast Company*, Omada has raised $126.5 million in six rounds of financing.

"Composing" a Diabetes Program

Sean Duffy compares tech design to writing a symphony. He admits it sounds a bit outlandish, but as he explains it, the analogy works. "If you were Beethoven composing the *Fifth Symphony*, it would be very hard to do it with just the bassoonist in a way that's emotionally moving. You need to work with all the instruments to plan a great score. That's how we really think of design—it is the symphonic conduction of all the pieces that just create music that pulls people through," he explains.

In this case, the "instruments" are a pedometer and a cellular-enabled scale sent to each Omada participant, who also receives the online curriculum, personalized coaching and connection to support groups. Participants are divided into groups of 18 to 24 based on their location, age and other factors. Each group is assigned an online coach. Participants share data with their coach and with each other. The Omada program unlocks new lessons weekly and the coaches are available to answer questions via text, email or phone. Using their smartphones, users can take a photo of their meals and send it to their coach for review, or use the program's app to enter simple descriptions of their meals.

Although individuals can sign up online, Omada is primarily available to employers, health plans and payers who offer the service to eligible employees and beneficiaries as a preventive benefit. Omada gets reimbursed based on how well people achieve and maintain their goals.

Omada is not just another health app. It is a comprehensive program that includes several components that have to operate in tandem and that Duffy believes are vital to its success. "You can't just mail someone a scale and show them a chart. You can't just access a coach on the phone or through messaging. You can't just give someone the curriculum. You couldn't just put people on a group messaging board. You need to lay it all out on the same time line," he says.

Since its founding, Omada has enrolled more than 110,000 participants in all 50 states. The median age of an Omada user is 46 years old. Peer-reviewed published studies have shown that Omada can work as well or better at helping people maintain weight loss and control blood sugar than conventional diabetes prevention programs.

You may think that a digital coaching program that requires tracking would be great for younger adults, but not a good fit for older people, and you'd be wrong. In reality, older adults do better than younger people in the face-to-face National DDP, and the same holds true for Omada's digital version. In a study published in October 2016 in *PLOS ONE,* researchers looked at data on more than 1,100 overweight or obese adults aged 65 or older who were at high risk for diabetes or heart disease. The subjects were enrolled in Omada's program. Twenty-six weeks into the program, participants had lost on average 6.8% of their body weight and 89% had completed nine or more of the 16 weekly lessons.

The researchers concluded that if the participants sustained their weight loss and other improvements, it could reduce their healthcare costs by more than $13,000 over the next 10 years; reduce the risk of developing diabetes by up to 41% for people who are prediabetic; and reduce the risk for stroke by 15% in those at risk for CVD over five years.

In a second study, reported in the January 2017 issue of the *Journal of Aging and Health,* researchers followed 501 patients at high risk of developing diabetes, median age 68.8 years old. These participants were enrolled in the Omada Diabetes Prevention Program through Humana Medicare Advantage insurance. A year after starting the program, participants had lost an average of more than 13 pounds from an average initial weight of 208, or about 7.5% of their initial bodyweight. Participants also showed, on average, a −0.14% decrease in their HbA1C and a 7.08 mg/dL reduction in total cholesterol. The researchers noted, "This level of weight loss exceeds the benchmark set by the CDC's National Diabetes Prevention Program, which aims for a 5% reduction in weight at 6 months and 12 months."

Omada also enables users to connect to each other, sharing data and offering support. Interestingly, participants in the program not only reported better health metrics, they reported improvements in well-being, depression symptoms and self-care.

Omada may be a high-tech program, but it strives to be very easy to use. For example, all the tech components come automatically synced to the user's online account. Unlike many commercial smart scales, the Omada scale is embedded with a cellular chip, so there is no need for users to pair it with Bluetooth or Wi-Fi.

Duffy notes that he didn't dumb down his tech so that older people could use it. Nor does he feel that age is a factor in technology design. "When I'm on panels or making presentations, people always ask me, 'Well, can seniors use your technology?' We believe that the question's flipped. Good technology design is about creating tools that *anybody* can use," he says. "I think the products that can have the biggest impact need to be really simple and intuitive and the details need to be ironed out, and that's true for anybody."

There are many reasons I admire Omada and Sean Duffy, but we see eye-to-eye on design, as evidenced by this comment. So much technology we ask people to use has major design flaws. There are nuances, but in general, well-designed, engaging software can transcend many demographic groups. Omada is clever because the company has designed its tools to be easy-to-get and easy-to-use. It is hard enough to employ the self-discipline required to correct insulin resistance, so they wisely made the first steps easy.

Omada did detect some interesting differences in how older users approached their material versus younger program participants. Initially older users were a bit more timid about exploring new lessons ahead of time or taking advantage of some of the added features, like online chats. But with a bit of prodding in the form of added instruction, Duffy notes they not only engaged, but did so at higher rates than younger users. "I think this really shows that there's need for a few extra teaching moments when you open up new elements of a program. Once you do that, you can get really good engagement."

In particular, Duffy says, older users are much more socially oriented than younger ones. "We see that older individuals have a higher group engagement rate. They'll get on a group-oriented chat more often. I think it delivers this secondary benefit, connection to a neat social community. You may be retired, have a little bit more time on your hands. It's a nice way to engage with other people."

From the get-go, Omada has been conducting clinical trials to move acceptance for digital therapies, which Duffy says still maintain "underdog" status in the medical community. "When we started, there was very little evidence that digital programs had any impact. We needed to create that on our own, to promote digital coaching as a counterpart to in-person coaching. Right now, we have seven publications, and we're going to very quickly double that number to show clinical impact of the other outcomes our program may be achieving, but we just aren't yet in the peer-reviewed literature."

The "other outcomes" include improvement in metrics like blood lipids and inflammatory markers, but also a deeper dive into emotional issues, like loneliness and well-being. Says Duffy, "Loneliness is a big problem for older people and can lead to poor health outcomes. Can our program for seniors improve that? What about stress and resilience? We hypothesize, based on the way that people are engaging, that, 'Yes, it's possible that there are benefits in this area.'" To my mind, companies like Omada will do well if they create easy-to-use technology, engaging programs and inspiring coaching.

Relationship Building

Iora Health is a Boston-based primary care startup, launched in 2010. It describes itself as a company that is building "a radically new model of healthcare delivery from the ground up." Iora is very much the vision of its founder, Rushika Fernandopulle, MD, MPP, who didn't want to just reform healthcare, but to invent "a whole new operating system for healthcare." And he wanted to build it especially for high-risk patients who needed the most help, and who, he believed, were badly served by the existing system.

"Most of US healthcare is built on transactions and incentives," Fernandopulle explains. "One of our premises is that that approach hasn't worked. What we're aiming to do is to get rid of those transactions and focus on relationships."

In a January 11, 2014 *New Yorker* profile of what he called "stats-and-stethoscope upstarts," physician-author Atul Gawande, MD, MPH, wrote about one of Iora's first medical offices in Atlantic City run by Fernandopulle. It was part of an article on novel approaches to what the healthcare industry refers to as its "super utilizers," typically older, sicker patients who are the most expensive to the system, often because they fall between the cracks.

The article also featured Timothy G. Ferris, MD, MPH, chairman and CEO of the Massachusetts General Physicians Organization—and my colleague—who was the coordinator of a successful Medicare demonstration program that focused on caring for chronically high-cost patients, providing timely intervention when needed. Within three years, under Tim's leadership, the program met its target savings of 5% by reducing hospital stays and emergency department visits.

Gawande wrote, "We've been looking to Washington to find out how health-care reform will happen. But people like these are its real leaders."

Over the past few years, Iora has proven that making investments in wellness can pay off fairly quickly in terms of reducing the cost of caring for high-risk populations, without skimping on quality. It is free from the fee-for-service model that is driving up costs: Iora doctors are paid a flat fee. It offers a team-based practice—each patient is assigned to a doctor or nurse-practitioner, behavioral health specialist and health coach.

"Our model isn't for everyone," Fernandopulle notes. "We look for doctors who say, 'This is exactly how I want to practice medicine.'"

The company's stated mission is "restoring humanity to healthcare" and it prides itself on providing intensely personalized service to its patients. When a new patient joins the practice, he or she sits down with a coach and works out an individual plan. "They do it together. The coaches don't say, 'Eat better and get more exercise.' The coach will ask, 'What do you like to do? Do you like biking? Do you like walking?' and they'll build a program around that," Fernandopulle says. "When they're done, they don't dismiss the patient and say, 'OK now go off and take a walk.' No, they do intense follow-up. Our coaches hold their patients accountable. They hold their hands if they need that kind of support, or they kick their butts if that works better. They'll engage them in groups; they'll take someone shopping to show him how to pick out the right food. What we do is very personalized based on who we are treating."

To a large extent, Iora's proprietary technology—a very sophisticated, personalized form of analytics—has made this personalization possible. Michael Greeley of Flare Capital Partners, whom I quoted earlier, is an investor in Iora. Greeley notes, "Iora invests in novel technologies, analytics, novel communication platforms, messaging and so on. They're prepared to make those investments because their return is pretty immediate. They're doing at-risk care providing and their outcomes are dramatic."

Using the company's software, Iora coaches can keep close tabs on their patients; the company calls this "storytelling population health management." The medical staff and health coaches are able to access information about patient populations based on specific criteria. For example, a coach can search for patients who have blood pressure readings that are still too high despite treatment and receive a list of patients in that category. Coaches can use the data to identify patients who may require extra attention; having access to this information enables the doctors and the coaches to focus on patients who need the most help.

"Our philosophy is, you reach out to the patient any way that works, using all types of technology and human engagement," Fernandopulle explains. The Iora model is compelling for many reasons, chief among them the true patient-centeredness. I find it interesting that they recruit MDs by telling them that they get to practice the way they wish they could, but that the approach is very patient-focused. Fernandopulle deserves enormous credit for daring to launch a company based on the simple notion that care should "just make sense."

Although many health coaches are yoga instructors, dietitians or from other areas of health and wellness, this is not a requirement for becoming a coach. What's required is a passion for the company's mission. As Fernandopulle says, "They're people who are picked for their empathy, who can work with patients in a longitudinal way to try and engage them."

Iora also offers patients access to Chirp, its proprietary collaborative care platform that enables patients to keep track of all of their health information in one place, as well as exchange emails or texts with their doctors. Chirp is designed for a computer or smartphone.

Focus on the Underserved

Fernandopulle says that the company is now increasing its focus on the most underserved and complex patients—especially people aged 65 years and older on Medicare.

As of Spring 2017, Iora Primary Care included 18 primary care practices designed specifically for patients aged 65 and older. They are scattered around the country, with two located in the Boston area through Tufts Health Plan Medicare Preferred HMO plans and Tufts Health Plan Senior Care Options plan. Locations in Arizona, Colorado and Washington State are through the Humana Medicare Advantage insurance plan. Each facility includes a gerontologist as well as health coaches to work individually with patients. Iora also offers older adults yoga classes, nutrition guidance, a diabetes club and other services depending on the patient's needs.

Iora has contracts with Medicare Advantage primarily through Humana and Tufts. In an era of cost cutting, Iora's business model seems improbable: It charges the insurer $100 per person per month, double the customary fee charged to Medicare for primary care. The monthly fee, however, also covers coaching and other programs offered by Iora, including the exercise classes. Despite the higher upfront cost, Iora produces savings for Medicare. The typical Medicare patient costs the system around $12,000 annually; the average Iora Medicare Advantage patient costs around 20% less. The savings comes from fewer hospitalizations and fewer visits to specialists. Although Iora will refer patients to a specialist if they need to see one, Fernandopulle says their approach has shown that better management of patients—and more focus on the individual needs of each patient—can reduce the need for specialists.

According to Fernandopulle, "The paradigm right now in US healthcare, and particularly in Medicare, is that you have a cardiologist managing your hypertension, an endocrinologist managing your diabetes, a pulmonologist managing your COPD and so on. On top of that, you may be seeing a cognitive specialist every now and then. That is a completely broken system, because all of these things are connected. If you try to isolate one from the other, it won't work. We say, 'We will take care of you, and we will get the help we need, when we need it, but we will take care of you, period.' That's a different way to look at it."

In June 2004, as the first executive director of the Harvard University Interfaculty Program for Health Systems Improvement, Fernandopulle opened his first primary care practice just outside of Boston, where he began to design the model of care that would later become Iora Health. He included innovative features like health coaches, email and targeting, and working more closely with the sickest and least compliant patients. His practice didn't last, a failure that Fernandopulle attributes to being ahead of its time and having to overcome too many hurdles created by forces not interested in supporting its radical new style of delivering health.

Although Iora is an innovator in the use of analytics and other forms of health tech, Fernandopulle is adamant that technology alone is not a panacea for the healthcare crisis. He feels strongly that there is a dire need to change the culture of healthcare and that the first step is to become a truly patient-centric system. He looks to successful consumer companies, like Zappos, Southwest Airlines and Ritz-Carlton as models for how healthcare providers should treat their patients. (Tony Hsieh, CEO of Zappos, is an early Iora investor and has served on its Advisory Board.)

Fernandopulle asserts that, "It's things like allowing consumers to interact with us in the way that they want to, not the way we want to. In every other part of the economy, businesses interact with people they deal with by email, by text message, by phone, by video. It's ridiculous that in healthcare we don't do that, and it's because of our hang-ups, not theirs. We make all sorts of excuses and blame HIPAA and other stuff, but they are just excuses from people who don't want to change. At Iora, we build around the notion that the medical record belongs to the patient. That's what the law says, but most of the time in healthcare, we make it very difficult for patients to access that information. We hide stuff from them and we say that we're "trying to protect them," but it's again one of the many excuses that people give who don't want to change the system."

Fernandopulle warns that healthcare companies that don't change will become obsolete. "We have all these great technologies, like texting, emails, video chats and Fitbits. We should use these tools as part of the health system—not as opposition to it. I think, unfortunately, most of the current healthcare delivery systems and players are unwilling or unable to make that transition. I think the real answer is going to be that, at some point, they're going to need to either figure out how to make the transition or get the hell out of the way. That's just what happens."

The fact that Iora can reduce Medicare costs per patient by 20% is significant. According to the US Department of Health & Human Services, in FY 2017, gross current law spending on Medicare benefits will total $709.4 billion. If you cut 20% of the total cost of care for each patient, just imagine the savings! And you do it by keeping people healthy.

Investors are enthusiastic about the Iora model. The company raised $75 million in 2016, which it plans to use to drive expansion and improve efficiencies, according to a press release announcing the financing. The Singapore-based investment firm Temasek led the funding round, with additional participation from Iora's existing investors. This is in addition to the $62 million the company has raised since its launch in 2010.

Can a Magic Picture Frame Rescue Healthcare?

In earlier chapters, I noted the lower usage of health tech among older adults of advanced age, precisely the group that could benefit the most from support. Care.coach is a Millbrae, California–based startup that is using a combination of high tech and human touch to improve self-management of chronic conditions among older adults. On its website, care.coach pitches itself as an "engagement and care coordination system" that enables providers to better manage their most complex patients over the care continuum. Care.coach is designed for use in homes as well as in hospitals.

"In the community, our typical patients are in their late 70s and have multiple chronic conditions. They may have Type 2 diabetes, many have been in and out of hospitals for heart failure and they may also have COPD," explains Victor Wang, CEO of care.coach. "They often have limited family support. They are generally not tech savvy. Few are using Google to research their health, or are on Facebook. And many are living alone."

Wang's company is directing its efforts precisely to the hard-to-reach older person who has been overlooked by health technology, and who requires significant care. These are the folks who may be overwhelmed by the task of managing their condition and end up being hospitalized for a problem that could have been prevented with the right intervention. This is a situation that is ripe for technological solutions.

A 2016 study published in *JAMA* found, "Digital health is not reaching most seniors and is associated with socioeconomic disparities, raising concern about its ability to improve quality, cost, and safety of their health care. Future innovations should focus on usability, adherence, and scalability to improve the reach and effectiveness of digital health for seniors."

Earlier, I wrote about how poor technology design can create an enormous barrier for older people. Care.coach is proving that older adults—even those who may be technologically challenged by today's standards—can benefit from the right kind of health tech. It is a step in the right direction.

The care.coach platform is a tablet-based service platform that Wang describes as a "magic picture frame," an interactive screen that is installed in the home or at a hospital bedside. It enables patients to interact with an avatar, a companion in the form of a virtual dog or cat depending on their preference, which provides real-time support. It requires absolutely no effort on the part of the user; after it is delivered to the home, you plug it in and it starts talking. There is no need to ever charge it or sync it with other devices. Similar to other successful technologies for older adults, the care.coach tech is effortless on the part of the user. The Omada Health program is another example of this approach.

Care.coach is not completely automated; it is a combination of smart AI and human intervention. The software automates chronic disease self-management and is programmed to help each patient follow a specific at-home protocol depending on his or her medical condition. For example, a patient with heart failure may be reminded to report on his weight daily to see if there is fluid build-up or to prop his legs up when he sits down to prevent blood from pooling in his extremities. Or a patient on a strict diet will be given pre-programmed tips on how to plan meals. Patients can also receive guidance and encouragement on sticking to their exercise routines or rehab programs.

What makes this virtual pet even more lovable—and feel real— are the real humans behind it. A globally distributed team of specially trained human health advocates is monitoring the video-audio stream. At any time, day or night, they can hear, see and talk to the users.

Working from home, generally in the Philippines or Latin America, the English (and Spanish) speaking health advocates are watching multiple screens simultaneously and are ready to intercede if they spot a problem or have to answer a question. The interactions with the advocates, through the pet avatar, form a strong bond between the patients and their screen pets.

Pet owners tend to anthropomorphize their pets. We talk to them like they are human and we endow them with humanlike emotions. So it's not surprising that people would respond positively to a virtual pet that can carry on a humanlike conversation (thanks to the humans behind the curtain) and that has the advantage of knowing a great deal about them. The avatar can talk with them about their families and their daily routines, and get them to open up about anything bothering them. This combination of human and software is going to be a recurring feature in successful companies and strategies for dealing with the increased demand that aging baby boomers put on the system. Many things can be outsourced to software, but having a person in the loop, if needed, will be key.

The care.coach service is available 24/7, with many proactive check-ins throughout the day, but the virtual pet can be seen to nap frequently, whenever the attention of a health advocate is not required. The screen can also go dark for patients who may be bothered by the glow of the backlight at night. The software alerts the human health advocate team when it senses movement or noise, potentially prompting a check-in. If the patient wants to chat, petting the avatar is sure to wake it up.

A Digital Home Companion

Nearly all of the care.coach patients living at home are taking multiple medications and many must manage these medications on their own. The pet avatar not only reminds the patients to take their medication on time, but can also observe them doing it. For some patients with memory issues, this is a very important feature. It also provides someone to talk to if the patient feels lonely, any time of the day or night. The digital dog or cat can deliver messages from family members, display family photos or even play games. If the patient shows any signs of trouble, is incoherent, doesn't take his medication or seems sick, the avatar can alert a healthcare provider or family member.

Care.coach, Wang's first startup, began as GeriJoy, an app developed in 2012 to "bring joy to geriatrics." The inspiration for the company came from Wang's grandmother, who the Wang family left behind when they moved from Taiwan to Canada when he was a young boy. Feeling socially isolated, his grandmother became very depressed and suicidal, forcing his mother to return to Taiwan for a year to help her out. When Wang was getting his master's degree at MIT, he researched human-machine interaction for NASA. He realized that the same principle of teleoperation that is used on the International Space Station could be useful in connecting families to older relatives living in far off places.

Care.coach promotes self-care by providing in-the-moment counseling and encouragement to people living at home who may be feeling lonely and discouraged. Care.coach is also being marketed to hospitals as a tool to provide better patient care, reduce costs and improve outcomes. Similar to its role in the home, care.coach can serve as another set of eyes and another friendly face for hospital staff who can't be everywhere all the time. Care.coach can help engage patients and alert hospital personnel to potential problems that can lead to longer hospitalizations, rehospitalizations and poorer outcomes.

A Companion at the Hospital

Wang notes that hospitals can be very unsettling places for older adults, who may suddenly find themselves in a completely unfamiliar setting, on new medications and just plain disoriented or even frightened. Some studies suggest that one-third to one-half of hospitalized elderly patients suffer from some form of delirium, which makes them vulnerable to other problems, like falls and accidents.

The one-on-one relationship interaction between the patient and avatar is especially important in helping to detect changes in cognitive function that may go unnoticed until a problem arises. The human behind the avatar can periodically administer the Confusion Assessment Method (CAM) to identify delirium and distinguish it from confusion or other signs of cognitive decline. "CAM is a checklist that involves observing the patient's ability to pay attention and respond to a series of interactions. These interactions can take the form of a few questions specifically asked to check their cognitive, memory or attentional function, for example, as part of a brain game that the avatar administers. Or it could just be a series of social interactions, like when the avatar asks, 'How was breakfast?' or 'Would you like to hear a song?' If we discover that there's a problem, we report it to the nursing station," Wang says.

Besides early detection and awareness of delirium, certain kinds of cognitive stimulation, particularly what's called reorientation, has been shown to help reduce the risk of developing delirium. The avatar helps to reorient patients to time, place and purpose, for example, by asking for help to read a clock and figure out what time of day it is or by asking if the lighting is dim enough for the patient to go to sleep comfortably at night. Wang adds that care.coach can engage patients by playing online versions of TV game shows like *Jeopardy* or *The Price Is Right*, providing some stimulation that is both familiar and fun for the older patients.

Keeping tabs on cognitive function is not just for the patient's mental well-being, because research shows that an episode of delirium results in an average increase in length of stay of 7.78 days, reducing the hospital's capacity to serve new patients, while increasing cost of care for that patient by $60,000 over the following year. Often delirium results in accidents like falls, costly to both the patient and provider. Each year, 700,000 patients suffer a fall while they are in the hospital. Each incident can extend the hospital stay by six to 12 days, adding to the cost of care. Studies in hospital settings have shown that care.coach can produce significant reductions in patient falls and delerium.

In "The Use of an Avatar Virtual Service Animal to Improve Hospital Outcomes in Older Adults," an abstract presented before the Gerontological Society of America's 69th Annual Scientific Meeting in New Orleans in November 2016, researchers noted, "Through preventive exercise, just-in-time care coordination, early detection, etc., the care.coach avatar platform can mitigate the risk posed by falls." The study also showed statistically significant mitigation of both delirium and loneliness.

Hospitals and senior care facilities go to great lengths to try to prevent falls and other accidents. Some put sensors in or around a bed to detect if a high-risk patient tries to get up on his own. Wang feels that the care.coach approach is more effective because, instead of waiting to intervene as a patient is headed for an accident, the avatar engages the patient so that it can monitor for signs of trouble. "We offer a proactive solution—other solutions are passive and reactionary," says Wang. "Bed sensors can tell when somebody is getting out of bed or has crossed a boundary on the side of the bed, but by the time the busy hospital staff can respond to the alert, the patient may already be on the floor."

Often, patients are put in restraints in their beds, which can increase their anxiety and upset their families, while decreasing key performance indicators for the hospital. In some cases, a hospital or care facility may hire "patient sitters" to literally sit next to a patient to catch the patient trying to get out of bed and thereby prevent a fall. Wang notes that this is a very expensive solution that research shows does not work well. "A typical hospital unit with 30 beds may have two bedside sitters at any time. That can cost about $20,000 a month. In theory, they're supposed to be engaging the patient and trying to prevent falls and delirium. But because the job frequently entails long periods of boredom—you have to let the patient rest, and even when the patient is alert, conversing with a high-risk, frail patient is often challenging at best—patient sitters are often found looking at their cell phones or have dozed off at the beside."

And sometimes patients fall because they're too weak to get out of bed on their own to use the bathroom, but are reluctant to ask for help. While 50% of all falls in the hospital occur on trips to the bathroom or within the bathroom itself, Wang ways that this is a particularly common problem among male patients. "Patients don't push the call button and they just try to get up on their own even though they were told not to. That's how a lot of falls happen."

Aware of this problem, the care.coach avatar can ask men leading questions like, 'Oh, are you comfortable right now?' And then if they say, 'Not really,' we can use that as an opportunity to ask, 'Oh, do you need to go to the bathroom soon?' And then we just get them help so they never actually have to ask for someone to help them."

Like Omada, care.coach has found the right mix of human intervention to technology. As Wang notes above, there are times when people *prefer* confiding something to an onscreen avatar, especially if it is something they are embarrassed about. But there are also times when human interaction is essential—and the right technology allows for both.

◆ ◆ ◆

STEPPING UP TO FITBIT

The ultimate goal of proactive health is getting people to step up to the plate to maintain their own health and wellness. It may be a phenomenon that we see only among the "worried well" and perhaps not among the people who may need it the most, but it's still a move in the right direction. There are millions of Americans who are taking the first step by wearing activity trackers to promote a healthy lifestyle. Although some brands of trackers are clearly going after the young and athletic, Fitbit is reaching out to people of all ages. It is also moving into healthcare.

Launched in early 2007 by James Park (CEO) and Eric Friedman (CTO), Fitbit went public in 2015. And in October 2016, Park told CNBC's Jim Cramer that Fitbit is "on the cusp of transitioning the mission and purpose of our company from a consumer electronics company to a digital healthcare company."

This is an exciting vision. If we think about activity as a new vital sign, you can envision this becoming a standard health measure in line with blood pressure, cholesterol levels and so on. I could even see us recalculating the cardiac risk index by blending activity into the equation.

In December 2016, Fitbit moved closer to achieving its goal of becoming a "digital healthcare company," by collaborating with Medtronic, a medical technology company that includes among its offerings continuous glucose monitoring (CGM) products and insulin pumps. Their first joint project was integrating Fitbit activity data into Medtronic's iPro2 myLog app, which enables patients with Type 2 diabetes to capture activity information that they can view in context with variability in their glucose levels. This is a terrific first step, as it is well known that the two major variables in glucose regulation in Type 2 diabetes are activity and diet. A doctor can tell a patient over and over again that increasing activity can help better control glucose levels, but actually seeing it happen for yourself makes it more real.

That said, the path from engaging the intrinsically motivated health enthusiast (Fitbit's current target customer) to the sedentary individual with two or more chronic illnesses (the target customer from a healthcare provider perspective) will be circuitous and take the company from its core competency of measurement into the much more complicated land of engagement.

The first popular digital tracker to reach the mainstream, Fitbit has 23.2 million active users, based on the latest figures available. It is the "Kleenex" of the digital health industry. Fitbit offers a suite of wearables that monitor daily activity, calories burned, sleep, heart rate and VO2 max (the maximum volume of oxygen that an athlete can use). Depending on the device, Fitbit also measures heart rate variability (the beat-to-beat changes in your heart rate). Last June, Fitbit announced that it was developing a device to detect sleep apnea, which is currently being tested in sleep labs.

The company's later wristbands, like Charge2 and Alta HR, and its smartwatch Blaze, have more bells and whistles than the early clip-ons, but all Fitbit trackers provide real-time feedback to users. Recently, Fitbit acquired Pebble and Vector, two smartwatch startups. Fitbit's Aria Wi-Fi Smart Scale is classified as a medical device by the FDA; It tracks weight, body mass index (BMI), lean mass and body fat percentage.

According to Fitbit, its data can help drive more informed patient-provider interactions. Fitbit is connected to leading electronic health record systems including Cerner, Epic and eClinicalWorks. The San Francisco–based company also provides a web

API (an application programming interface) for accessing data from its products, meaning that as long as a device or program is in compliance with Fitbit's API Terms of Use, anyone can develop an application to connect to Fitbit.

In May 2017, Fitbit announced that it had combined its Group Health and Digital Health operations to create Fitbit Health Solutions. Its new Health Solutions team focuses on developing health and wellness tools to help increase engagement, improve health outcomes and drive a positive return for employers, health plans and hospitals. As of early 2017, more than 2.6 million Fitbit users, including employees at 70 of the Fortune 500 companies, have connected their data into population health and health management platforms.

At CES 2017, the global consumer electronics and consumer technology tradeshow that takes place every January in Las Vegas, Fitbit announced it was adding new software and more social networking features that would allow for more interaction between users, notices about sponsored fitness events and tips from the company. According to Fitbit, users who have one or more Fitbit friends take about 700 more steps daily than those who don't. The company is also planning an expansion of FitStar, its personal trainer app that provides customized workout programs based on a person's Fitbit activity.

Like all wearables, Fitbit has not been able to retain users 100% of the time (studies show that up to half of all people who try any brand of tracker stop using it within six months). At CES, Fitbit CEO Park said, based on the latest figures available, "72% of the people who bought a device in 2015 were still actively using it at the end of the year." If that's the case, Fitbit is doing better than many other companies in this space.

But Fitbit's success up until now has more to do with tapping into the public's desire to stay well and vital than manage disease. In that respect, the company has nailed the "make it about life" part of consumer engagement.

Although the company doesn't break down users by age, anecdotally at least it appears as if it has a greater share of older users than its competitors. And unlike some of its competitors, Fitbit doesn't seem to be going after only the hard body, young millennials. A recent Fitbit commercial featured an older man who had been given a Fitbit Charge2 by his young-adult daughter. Not only did the dad begin working out, but he also began incorporating healthier eating into his life, as demonstrated by his drinking a green-colored vegetable smoothie. The commercial culminated with the father (looking svelte in a tuxedo) standing with his daughter at her wedding.

This commercial is spot-on in that it did not focus on illness, and it had an aspirational message: If you track your health, you will be around long enough to enjoy the good things in life. That's certainly a message that resonates with me, and I suspect with lots of other men and women of a certain age. It follows the strategies I outlined earlier about making health addictive, or "sticky."

Adam Pellegrini joined Fitbit in Fall 2016 and became the general manager of Fitbit Health Solutions in early 2017. Pellegrini came to Fitbit from Walgreen's Boots Alliance, where he was vice president of Digital Health. There, his team led the largest retail mHealth integration of more than one million connected devices via Walgreen's Balance Rewards program, which rewards customers for making healthy choices. I have known and respected Adam for some time. His imprint on Walgreens was very evident and has lasted beyond his tenure there.

Pellegrini says he has long admired Fitbit's ability to reach people of all ages and from all walks of life, something that is very difficult to achieve in healthcare. He attributes Fitbit's success to the fact that "there is no stigma attached to a Fitbit," because it's not associated with any particular illness, nor is it something sick people do.

"A Fitbit is for all ages, for everyone who has their own personal health and wellness goals, so this is not a device made for one specific population to manage their health," Pellegrini explains. "This is not a device for one specific population to manage Alzheimer's, or for one specific population to manage diabetes. Wearing a Fitbit is a badge that says, 'I consider my health and wellness very important to me. It's not about a condition or a disease, but it's about me as a person.'"

Pellegrini also feels the device will facilitate a better relationship between patients and providers. "A lot of people look at the Medtronic collaboration as being about enabling consumers to see both sets of data together and make the correlation on their own," Pellegrini explains. "But that's not what makes this powerful. Now the provider gets to see the physical activity, the behavioral data, sleep data and food data along with the Medtronic CGM (continuous glucose monitor). Now the provider can look at both data sources together and actually educate the patient on how physical activity and nutrition impact blood glucose levels. To me, that's a very powerful story to tell."

Pellegrini notes that although consumers can do a lot for themselves, the physician is the primary source of trusted information for patients, especially for the tens of millions of people who are managing diabetes. Many of these patients would use a tracker if their physicians recommended it. "As the physician becomes more comfortable educating a patient using both Fitbit data and

Medtronic data, which can now be viewed together, I think that's where providers will really start seeing the value of Fitbit, as well as other clinical data working together," Pellegrini adds.

Pellegrini says he has a "personal mandate" to really make it easier for healthcare systems to work with Fitbit, a trend that is already happening.

According to Pellegrini, some providers are taking it a step further, "We're already seeing hospitals actually integrating Fitbit into their care management systems—their dashboards—to include the Aria scale for congestive heart failure remote monitoring. But we have not yet created those really seamless ways to make it part of the workflow, and that's the first order of business. Otherwise we're just making work for them."

Until we can make it as easy for doctors and provider organizations to order a home-monitoring solution as it is to ask a nurse to call in to check on the patient, adoption will be low. We have to make the technology dead simple to order, to send the data and to have the data completely integrated into clinician work flow, not to mention have it reimbursed. Folks are working on all of these issues and I know it will happen.

CHAPTER 7

Putting the "Well" Back into Well-being

"There are very few people designing products for older adults who are focused on the fun, joy and happiness side of aging."
—TED FISCHER, VICE PRESIDENT, BUSINESS DEVELOPMENT, HASBRO, INC.

"I challenge tech developers to explore ways tech can help people achieve a higher sense of meaning and purpose. This could help people, in a great many ways, to improve both their psychological and physical health."
—ERIC S. KIM, PhD, RESEARCH FELLOW, HARVARD T.H. CHAN SCHOOL OF PUBLIC HEALTH AND SUBJECT MATTER SPECIALIST, AARP/AGE UK's GLOBAL COUNCIL ON BRAIN HEALTH

Hasbro's Ted Fischer and Harvard's Eric S. Kim are using words that you don't often hear in connection with health technology. Happiness. Meaning. Purpose. You may wonder, what does this have to do with gathering data and feedback loops? The fact is, health technology is not just a means of measuring key metrics and spitting back commands; it is a natural for enhancing social connections and creating motivation around activity.

Although I run Partners Connected Health, I also treat patients in the dermatology clinic at Massachusetts General Hospital. I, too, have observed the importance of nonmedical influences on my patients, such as family, friendship or feeling passionate about a job or hobby. I have observed three predictors of longevity in my patients: Companionship, a sense of purpose and moderate physical activity. This is purely observational and nonscientific, but, in my experience, quite reproducible. Of course, there are other factors, such as diet or genetic predisposition, that clearly have an impact on longevity and I don't mean to short-change them. If anything, the attention has been paid more to these factors, which is why I simply want to call attention to these somewhat softer metrics.

In previous chapters, I've focused on the importance of maintaining an active lifestyle and regular exercise. In particular, I've highlighted tools—wearables like Fitbit—that help motivate people to stay on a healthy track. But in this chapter, I investigate the other two factors for successful aging—companionship and purpose—and the importance of things like social connections, optimism and having a "mission," something that motivates you to get up in the morning. These factors are critical for a full and meaningful life at any age, but especially for people in their later years, when they may be facing new challenges that are an inevitable part of aging.

There is an enormous opportunity for health-tech developers to move beyond the standard tools (calorie counting, measuring steps, medication reminders and the like) to something that may one day prove to be equally, if not even more, powerful. Here, I delve into research on the impact of optimism, meaning and purpose on the aging process. More to the point of this book, I also highlight some innovative ways of using technology to help people stay social, happy and engaged with the world at any age.

My collaborator, Dr. Charlotte Yeh, has heightened my awareness of the role these factors play in our health—what many in the past would dismiss as "soft science." I admit that I approached this topic with some wariness, for two reasons. First, it's not my area of specialty, although I am learning that, as someone who has treated patients for more than three decades, I have more experience in this area than I had realized. Well-being plays a major role in healing. Second, I am grounded in hard science—speculation and theorizing is fine, but show me the data! Toward that end, in recent years, researchers have been producing some very interesting data.

Studies have shown that social isolation, loneliness and living alone are an *even greater* risk factor for premature death among the elderly than smoking or obesity. This can have significant implications for the health-care system: Studies show that as many as 40% of older adults report feeling lonely. This isn't just a quality of life issue, it's a health issue. In two different widely publicized studies, researchers at Brigham Young University reported that social isolation was as significant a threat to longevity as obesity. In earlier studies, the same research group, headed by Julianne Holt-Lunstad, PhD, found that loneliness was the equivalent of smoking 15 cigarettes a day or being an alcoholic, in terms of mortality risk.

A 2016 study of 12 million Facebook users, led by University of California, San Diego, researchers William R. Hobbs, PhD, and James Fowler, PhD, found that people who had the most Facebook friends lived longer than those in the lowest 10% of Facebook friends. The authors did not suggest any cause or effect to their study, but given what we know about the health benefits of social engagement, it's not too big a leap to suggest social networks may offer a way to boost social interaction and maintain relationships.

The reality is, the most negative aspect of loneliness could be the impact it has on our behavior. In 2016, AARP did a survey among adults aged 18 and over, to understand the link between healthy behaviors and mental well-being. According to Charlotte Yeh, "The results were pretty dramatic. Those with the most friends had the highest number of healthy behaviors."

Another recent survey of older adults, conducted by the CareMore healthcare plan and delivery system, found that 20% reported feeling isolated from family and friends. In response, CareMore is offering a "Togetherness Program," which the company describes as "a first-of-its-kind clinical effort that will address the social challenges aging seniors face on a daily basis, which are not systematically diagnosed and discussed in clinical practice." What's interesting is that we're beginning to see loneliness being treated as if it were a chronic medical condition.

It stands to reason that if people have little motivation to get up in the morning, they will also have little motivation to take their medications, eat well, get enough exercise or reach out to others. If we don't first solve these social and emotional problems, we may not be able to solve the physical problems that result from an unhealthy and neglectful lifestyle.

A Population at Risk

The elderly population is at particular risk for social isolation. The death of a spouse—particularly among men who are accustomed to their wives running their "social calendar"—can result in depression and loneliness. So can the diminishing number of healthy or living friends, a sad reality of aging. Family connections can become frayed as children move far away, which means that many older adults don't get to see their kids or grandchildren on a regular basis. And at some point, even the most independent among us may have to turn in the car keys, which, depending on where we live, can be very isolating. (Yes, there will be a market for self-driving cars!)

Physical ailments can also interfere with social interaction, resulting in loneliness and isolation, which, in turn, can lead to more physical and mental deterioration. It becomes a vicious cycle. Hearing loss, the most common physical problem among the elderly, is a prime example of a physical condition that can lead to a downward spiral. According to the National Institute on Deafness and Other Communication Disorders, hearing loss impacts one in three people between the ages of 65 and 74, and nearly half of those 75 and older. There are volumes of studies that show a link between hearing loss and social isolation among older adults. Even moderate hearing loss can make it difficult to carry on a conversation, even in a quiet setting, but it can make it nearly impossible to do so in a crowded and loud room. If you can't hear or make yourself understood, why bother going to the party or out to dinner, or even to church?

I'm sure some of you are thinking that the solution is to give everyone a hearing aid, but that's not so simple. Hearing aids can help, but they're still far from perfect (especially in a crowded room) and only one in five older adults who need a hearing aid actually uses one. Some people shun them for fear that wearing a hearing aid will label them as "old." But there are also other obstacles to obtaining a hearing aid: In most cases, hearing aids are available only by Rx, they can be quite expensive and are usually not covered by Medicare. I wouldn't exactly call this making it easy for the consumer.

Hearing loss isn't just a social liability; it can lead to many serious, even life-threatening problems. The primary cause of hearing loss in the elderly is caused by damage or death of tiny hair cells in the inner ear. These cells are also instrumental in helping people maintain balance. That's how hearing loss (or the degeneration of this portion of the inner ear) increases the likelihood of falls. In turn, fear of falling can make people anxious about venturing out of the house, and that too can cause more social isolation. As I said, it's a vicious cycle.

Most alarmingly, hearing loss significantly increases the risk of developing dementia. Frank Lin, MD, PhD, and head of the Lin Research Group at Johns Hopkins, has led a number of studies on the impact of hearing loss on the physical and mental health of older adults. Lin's group found that people with mild hearing loss had double the risk of developing dementia in their lifetime; people with severe hearing loss were five times more likely to. Furthermore, Lin's research revealed that people with hearing loss lose more brain tissue as they age than those with normal hearing. Could social isolation—and lack of brain stimulation—be the reason why the brain is shrinking? Based on everything that we know about "brain aging" and the need to stay active and engaged, it's a reasonable hypothesis. Lin's group is working on new studies to determine whether hearing aids could reduce or prevent the increased risk for dementia among older adults.

Ultimately, technology may come to the rescue. We've heard a great deal about a new category of wearables called "hearables," personal sound amplifiers (with noise canceling capability) that will be intended for people of all ages. As I write this, Congress passed the Over-the-Counter Hearing Aid Act of 2017, which President Trump signed into law, making hearing aids available with an Rx for people with mild to moderate hearing loss. Given the need among the older population (and a growing need among younger people), over-the-counter hearables could be the next big thing. Hearables could also prove to be a major cure for loneliness, as well as a tool for sharpening the brain.

The Hard Facts about "Soft" Science

In this book, we've focused on the increase in lifespan over the past century, but there are pockets of the population that are not enjoying this newfound longevity. In 2015, Princeton University Professors Anne Case, PhD, and Nobel laureate Sir Angus Deaton, PhD, reported on a disturbing trend: The steady rise in death rates, since 1999, among middle-aged non-Hispanic white Americans. They attributed this decline in longevity to "the deaths of despair," from drugs, alcohol and suicide.

In "Mortality and morbidity in the 21st century," a paper that is part of the Spring 2017 edition of the *Brookings Papers on Economic Activity (BPEA)*, the researchers offered further explanation about this trend. In particular, they noted that the hardest hit group were working class whites who had a high school degree or less, and who were most likely to be unemployed, unmarried and childless. You could say that they lost their purpose in life. And, as a result, they were more likely to engage in unhealthy behaviors that cut life short, like alcohol and opiate abuse and smoking. They were also more likely to have mental health issues that often went untreated.

My point in mentioning this is that we can't have a discussion about improving outcomes and efficiencies in healthcare without factoring in and responding to the psychological and emotional state of people. If you ignore this "soft science" you will be sabotaging your own efforts. Studies have demonstrated that optimistic people, those who have a generalized expectation that good things will happen, live longer than those who don't. Furthermore, how we view the aging process itself is a major predictor of what the bean counters would call "outcomes."

Since the mid-1990s, Yale School of Public Health's Becca Levy, PhD, professor of Epidemiology (Social and Behavioral Sciences) and Psychology, has been exposing the toxic impact of ageism on health and longevity. In 2002, Levy's group reported in a study published in *The Journal of Personality and Social Psychology* that, based on personal interviews conducted up to 23 years earlier, older individuals with more positive self-perceptions of aging lived 7.5 years longer than those with less positive self-perceptions of aging.

In other words, if you have a negative view of aging, it will be a self-fulfilling prophecy. In 2009, Levy posited the stereotype embodiment theory (SET) as a theoretical model to explain how our beliefs about older people and aging can impact the aging process. She cites several reasons why perception of aging could impact health, including the fact that people who have a negative view of aging may not believe that engaging in healthy behaviors will reap any benefit for them.

In 2015, Levy's research group made headlines with two intriguing papers published in the journal *Psychology and Aging*. Levy and her colleagues used information collected by the Baltimore Longitudinal Study of Aging, which had assessed the participants' perceptions of aging decades before performing brain MRIs and brain autopsies. First, the MRIs revealed that people who had the most negative views of aging when they were younger had a greater decline in hippocampus volume as they aged. The hippocampus is a complex, important part of the brain and we can't say for sure what this correlation means, but hippocampal loss is associated with Alzheimer's disease. Second, the researchers examined brain autopsies of the same group. They found that people with the most negative stereotypes of aging also had a greater build-up of amyloid plaques and neurofibrillary tangles in their brains, two other characteristics of Alzheimer's disease. The researchers noted, "These findings suggest a new pathway to identifying mechanisms and potential interventions related to the pathology of Alzheimer's disease."

When interviewed after the brain studies became public, Levy hypothesized that people were so stressed out by their negative views on aging that, as they aged, they experienced the same kind of physical damage to the brain that is seen in people who have been living in very stressful situations.

Putting a Number on It

Harvard's Eric S. Kim is one of a growing number of researchers who are exploring the connection between "nonmedical" factors—like positive psychological functioning, perceptions of aging, social connections, emotional state and retirement status—that, early results suggest, have a significant impact on health. Kim is a research associate at the Harvard School of Public Health and also part of the Lee Kum Sheung Center for Health and Happiness at Harvard, launched in 2016 to "support the identification of psychological, social, and emotional strengths and assets that may protect against some diseases and enable people to enjoy longer, happier, and healthier lives."

Kim's interest in this topic stems back to his childhood: He noticed an interesting trend among some of his older relatives and parents' friends. Even if people were in good health when they retired from their jobs, they seemed to deteriorate rapidly postretirement. The exceptions were those who re-engaged in meaningful activities, like volunteering, caring for family members or starting an encore career—these people managed to stay vital and healthy. Kim speculated that there was a connection between health and retirement, but he wasn't sure what it was.

The answer came to him when, as an undergraduate psychology student at the University of Michigan, he read *Man's Search for Meaning*, psychiatrist-neurologist Viktor Frankl's moving memoir of his life in Nazi death camps. In his book, Frankl espoused his belief, based on his own experiences, about how having a purpose in life can enable people to survive even the most horrific conditions.

For Kim, Frankl's book filled in the blanks. As he recalls, "I realized that when people retire, they might lose their meaning in life, their purpose. I suspected that after retirement, many of them had stopped engaging in healthy activities that were keeping them well."

Kim was so intrigued by this revelation that he decided to devote his career to, as described on his academic website, researching "the different ways that people pursue the good life (e.g., through: purpose in life, personal growth, optimism, resilience, positive emotions) and how these pursuits influence various health behaviors and outcomes."

Kim defines *purpose* as having "a sense of meaning, a sense of direction and overarching goals." A number of studies headed by Kim have documented the critical role that purpose and positive psychological factors may play in promoting health.

"In our studies, higher purpose in life was longitudinally associated with a reduced risk of stroke, myocardial infarction, sleep disturbances and declines in physical functioning," Kim says. "We know that people who have a higher purpose in life engage in healthier behaviors. We have seen that when there is a drop in purpose, it appears as if it can be quite damaging, especially as people get older."

Kim was curious about the fact that fewer than half of all people over the age of 65 are up-to-date with core preventive services, like proper medical tests or flu shots. When he was doing his graduate work at the University of Michigan, he led several studies investigating the role that purpose in life may play in determining the likelihood of people taking advantage of preventive services. His team examined participants from the University of Michigan Health and Retirement Study (HRS), a large-scale longitudinal study supported by the National Institute on Aging and the Social Security Administration. Launched in 1992, the study has surveyed a comprehensive sample of Americans over the age of 50.

Starting in 2006, Kim's team tracked more than 7,100 respondents over six years. The researchers found that people who scored high on psychological tests for purpose in life were much more likely to take obtain several preventive screenings, including cholesterol tests, colonoscopies, mammograms, pap smears, prostate exams and flu shots.

And here is a statistic that will make those bean counters smile: Purpose in life was associated with fewer overall doctor visits and fewer overnight hospitalizations. Compared to people with the lowest purpose, people with the highest purpose make 32% fewer doctor visits and spend 61% fewer overnights in the hospital. That translates into significant cost savings.

The researchers concluded, "These results may facilitate the development of new strategies to increase use of preventive healthcare services and improve health, thereby offsetting the burden of rising healthcare costs in our aging society."

One of those strategies could be convincing some retired people to do volunteer work. In another study using HRS data, Kim's team found that people who had done volunteer work after retirement were more likely to take advantage of preventive healthcare services. Both men and women were more likely than nonvolunteers to receive cholesterol tests and flu shots; women were more likely to get mammograms and pap smears; and men more likely to get prostate exams.

How could factors like purpose and optimism influence his findings? Kim says there are three mechanisms that could be responsible:

First, as he initially suspected, these factors have a direct impact on behavior. People with higher purpose and optimism act in healthier ways. They want to stay around long enough to achieve their goals and aspirations. But Kim also notes that there are some intriguing randomized control studies that show that it's possible to induce positive emotions in people and, by doing so, trigger an improvement in behavior.

He cites one 2012 study that was published in the *Archives of Internal Medicine* (now called *JAMA Internal Medicine*) that followed some 240 patients recruited from the New York Presbyterian Hospital–Weill Cornell campus who had undergone coronary angioplasty. Within one year after the procedure, 20% of patients typically experienced new adverse events, but that risk can be reduced by 25% if they engage in physical activity. The researchers noted, " . . . however, physical activity is widely underused." In other words, it's hard to get people to stick to an exercise routine.

In this study, half of the group received behavioral interventions designed to encourage them to exercise, which included an educational workbook, a pedometer and a behavioral contract for a self-selected physical activity; the other half were given the same, along with an additional workbook chapter focusing on how to self-induce positive affect and self-affirmation; bi-monthly phone calls to induce positive affect and self-affirmation; and small, unexpected bi-monthly gifts in the mail. The second group were also urged to "think about things that make you feel good" and to engage in self-affirmation exercises when they didn't want to do their daily exercise, like thinking about "proud moments" in their lives. Both groups were also contacted bi-monthly for follow-up.

The results, as Kim says, were pretty amazing. "The patients [in the second group] who participated in the counseling calls were 1.7 times more likely to attain their physician-recommended levels of physical activity within a year than those who did not. That's an example of the types of really intriguing studies that are coming out and illustrating that behavioral pathway."

In some ways this describes a lesson we've learned many times and that I've written about previously in *The Internet of Healthy Things*: That is, tracking activity and adding in a motivational program (in this case, the psychological tools described above) will result in increased physical activity.

What makes this study interesting is that it may give us a clue as to how a sense of purpose and positive thinking work to increase longevity. The connection with physical activity is also intriguing. Perhaps those of us with purpose and positive thinking are releasing beneficial hormones and chemicals into our bloodstream that decrease inflammation and lower stress. It goes back to the mind-body connection. I am impressed by how we keep learning how strong this connection really is and how it may influence systems we think of as purely physiologic, like the cardiovascular system.

The second pathway is that people who share high purpose, optimism and positive views of aging, have better coping mechanisms. "They have contingency plans worked out ahead of time. If Plan A fails, they go to Plan B or Plan C, which they had preplanned," Kim explains. "They seek more social support in times of stress and they actually disengage from goals that they think are unattainable, and all these kinds of things lead to reduced amounts of toxic stress, which, in turn, leads to better health."

The final pathway, according to Kim, is one that has been recently discovered—these kinds of emotional states may actually have a direct impact on our biology. "There is a really fascinating study from 2015 that was described in *Nature,* which showed that there's a physical structure linking the brain with our lymphatic system, which is interconnected with several systems in our body, including our immune system," he says.

The last pathway is particularly interesting because it suggests that positive emotion could have an impact that is independent of our behavior. "We need to study this more closely," Kim adds.

This brings Kim back to the topic that he chose for his life work: the study of meaning, purpose and optimism. Kim is fascinated by a concept that he read about in *The Blue Zones: Lessons for Living Longer From the People Who've Lived the Longest* by Dan Buettner. People who live on Okinawa, a "blue zone" where people routinely live to be 100-plus, use the term *ikigai,* which translates as "a reason for which you wake up in the morning."

"This reason for living isn't always large and grand in scope—although it is sometimes," Kim says. "For example, some people would say that their *ikigai* is tending a vegetable garden that helps feed their children and grandchildren. It's whatever gets them up in the morning with a sense of purpose. We need to do more research on this concept," Kim says.

This is all fascinating, but this book is about the role of technology in extending longevity. How does a concept like *ikigai* factor in? One way would be the gig economy—a lab or market focused on short-term or project work, often virtually, that allows flexibility and work-on-demand. With companies like TaskRabbit and Viatask, workers are able to create their own schedules and manage work-life balance in a way we've never imagined before. Many of the jobs offered on these sites are time-and-place-independent assignments. This is a perfect match for individuals who have the wisdom that only seasoning brings, but have physical constraints, or who simply want to work part time.

VR for Life Enhancement

"I think a big problem we're facing in the current aging paradigm is that health technology is all about life maintenance, not life enhancement. We think that virtual reality (VR) can actually change the paradigm," says Dennis Lally of Rendever, whom you met in Chapter 2.

Lally was working toward his MBA at MIT's Sloan School of Management when he met fellow student Reed Hayes. Lally had a strong interest in both healthcare and entrepreneurship; Hayes was fascinated by the potential of virtual reality and, at the time, was watching an aging family member struggle with social isolation and loneliness. Lally and Hayes decided to build a virtual reality platform to improve the aging process for older adults by providing cognitive stimulation and therapeutic virtual experiences.

VR has already been used in health settings to help people cope with PTSD, depression and pain management, among other medical and emotional issues, but not for our aging population. Yet, there is a great need for tools to help older adults manage life changes, like illness or having to leave their homes for assisted living. Studies show that older adults living in long-term-care facilities will often experience depression and isolation during their stay, a trend that Lally feels VR can help reverse. "We're using VR to prevent people from becoming socially isolated and depressed, and to keep them happy and healthy," he explains.

Today, Rendever works with several partners to build content for Samsung VR headsets and is developing its own proprietary content. The Rendever platform deviates somewhat from the standard VR system to make it work for people who may have cognitive or dexterity deficits. The designers found that older adults had difficulty manipulating the control pad that is embedded in the temple of the headset. Instead, the system is controlled by a tablet that can be guided by an activity director, caregiver or even another assisted living resident.

"Once we built the platform, we realized that VR can be very isolating, so we thought, 'What can we do to make it more social?' A lot of the problems we were trying to solve were around isolation and we didn't want to make that more of an issue. We created group-sync functionalities, so that multiple VR headsets can all be operated at the same time, so people can share in experiences."

The Rendever design team spent a great deal of time living alongside residents in adult communities and interviewing hundreds of them to better understand their needs. Lally was especially moved by the story of an older woman who, despite wearing a fall monitor while she was living at home, resisted pressing the emergency alert button after she slipped because she didn't want anyone to know that she had fallen. Why? "She didn't want to lose her independence," Lally explains. "She realized that the fall could lead to her being forced into a situation where she needed to move into a senior care community. It's stories like these that made me realize that younger people often make decisions for older people, not with them. So we also wanted to create a tool that gave people lots of choices and made them feel independent."

Although the VR experience is guided by the tablet operator, the users can choose among a large library of VR content, ranging from a tour of the Louvre to exploring US national parks, attending a concert or swimming with sharks. They can enjoy the experience solo or simultaneously with family and friends also wearing headsets.

Lally adds that a feature called "Family Moments" allows family members to use a 360-degree camera to film a wedding, graduation or other event that can be converted into a VR experience and uploaded onto a parent or grandparent's Rendever VR account.

Lally also noticed that the people he interacted with were often nostalgic for the past. "One of the first things we did was build some algorithms to put Google Street View into virtual reality. This allows people to go someplace that is meaningful to them, without actually having to ask a relative to drive them back to their old neighborhood. They can visit it on their own, anytime they want."

Lally admits that in the beginning, the team wondered how difficult it would be to get older adults to use this new technology. As it turned out, it wasn't a problem. "They love using VR; they see someone else using it and they want to try it."

Rendever's system can be found in communities around the country, where, according to Lally, residents have experienced a 40% increase in happiness scores. Lally says that Rendever is working with both Harvard and MIT's AgeLab to conduct studies to determine whether providing residents with a VR experience can actually change their behavior, in terms of making them more amenable to socializing and engaging in healthy behaviors.

"Because they're happy that they went on a virtual experience—attending a concert or a family party virtually—perhaps they may be more willing to partake in the therapy that the doctor prescribed," Lally says. "Or maybe they'll take their medication without arguing about it or be willing to go out and take a walk. If we have some initial data that says yes, then the next question is: How does it actually effect clinical outcomes and improve the overall health of these individuals? We need to do some clinical studies to answer these questions."

Virtual reality is in the earliest phases of development and adoption. An analogy would be the launch of Netscape Navigator in 1995. We were in awe of this new technology, where you pointed your mouse at a bit of underlined text and were transported to a whole different content area. Think of what the web has become today and you'll get a sense, by analogy, of the possibilities of VR. What I like about Rendever is that the company combines the fantasy aspects of VR with social connection, which tackles two problems at once—isolation and boredom.

Joy for All: A Game Changer

Chances are, you've played a game or with a toy that falls under the Hasbro, Inc., portfolio of brands, such as Transformers, Monopoly, Play-Doh, My Little Pony or Nerf. Recently this iconic Pawtucket, Rhode Island–based global play and entertainment company came up with a real game changer. In November 2015, Hasbro launched its Joy for All Companion Pets, designed to bring "comfort, companionship and fun to elder loved ones." Companion Pets are interactive, high-tech, cuddly friends that provide much of the fun of pet ownership without the hassle.

Hasbro isn't just selling a cool product—the company is selling well-being. It is targeting a vast market that has long been neglected in the game world: older adults. The concept has taken off. When the Joy for All brand first launched, its Companion Pets were sold on the JoyForAll.com website and with Amazon. Within nine months, the pets had been picked up by Walmart.com, Target.com, QVC and CVS.

Hasbro's first Joy for All Companion Pet was a cat offered in three different fur colors: silver, creamy white and orange tabby. Joy for All Companion Cats have built-in sensors that respond to motion and are covered in soft fur. They feature lifelike purring that you can hear and feel, thanks to a VibraPurr feature. The cats make 32 different sounds and have expressive eyes that can blink and look at you. Similar to real cats, they can be unpredictable and may roll over and meow as you interact with them.

As Ted Fischer, Hasbro's vice president of Business Development explains, "Cats never do what you want them to do when you want them to do it, so the play pattern of Companion Pets is also completely random. You may touch the sensor on the back and the cat may meow or it may not. It may purr or it may not. It may roll over, or not. It's not going to do the same thing and I think that's part of the fun of this interactive pet."

The Joy for All Companion Cat was received so well by the aging community that, in 2016, the company launched a Joy for All Companion Pet Golden Pup that has a simulated heartbeat that you can hear and feel. It can also turn its head and respond to sounds. The puppy is more active than the cat, but will calm down when you lay it down on your lap. "If you start petting the toy when it's on your lap, it stops acting like a playful puppy. When you quietly put your hand on its back, you can feel a faint heartbeat, like with a real dog. So you are both resting and it's very calming," Fischer says.

Although Hasbro does not make any therapeutic or health claims for its Companion Pets, the pets are being well-received in assisted living and long-term care facilities as a tool to stem loneliness and, in some cases, reduce anxiety, especially among dementia patients. Hasbro has donated Companion Pets to Meals on Wheels for the homebound elderly, because, as Fischer puts it, "they deal with loneliness and isolation on a daily basis."

The concept for Joy for All came about when Hasbro noticed through consumer reviews posted via online retailers that many of its products intended for children were actually being purchased by adult caregivers for aging loved ones. Hasbro recognized a void in the older adult market and decided to fill it.

Fischer, who joined Hasbro in early 2015, says the mandate of his group is "to think about how we would leverage Hasbro's many assets in new markets and new channels." He adds that "the health and wellness area just kept bubbling to the top in terms of opportunities to leverage our products and our brands."

As part of their research, Fischer and his team attended industry conferences on health and aging, but found it to be a "joyless" experience. "I know that there are a lot of necessary products out there for this market, but does it all have to be so grim? When we were walking through the exhibition halls, all I could think was, 'Gee, if these were the only products somebody brought into my home—if I was the intended user of these products—I would constantly be reminded of all the negative aspects of age and stage!' These products didn't exactly promote happiness," he recalls.

The Hasbro team also reached out to senior living communities and talked to staff and residents to learn more about what kind of product would bring "joy, fun and play" into their lives. They found some common themes; in particular, many residents told them how much they missed having a pet. "It was a great source of sadness for them because they had been very attached to their pets," Fischer says. "But they either weren't allowed to have a pet in the community or had to give up a pet because they could no longer care for it."

Fischer notes that designing products in health and wellness was a natural for Hasbro, because it tapped into the assets that the company already exceeded in. "We are very good at value engineering, the ability to do something with high quality for a lot lower cost. In this market, where products typically cost a lot, it is a great opportunity." In other words, Hasbro could produce products in this space that would be cheaper than the current offerings.

For example, Hasbro's Companion Cat retails for $99 and the Pup for $119. In contrast, there are other robotic pets on the market that have been used in care facilities, which are significantly more expensive. For example, the Paro advanced therapeutic robotic baby harp seal, developed by Japan–based AIST, is a Class II medical device that comes with a price tag of around $6,000. Paro has been used with memory and dementia patients in Japan and Europe, and as a substitute for a live pet for older adults who can no longer care for one.

Despite the fact that Hasbro has not made any health claims, the price makes it possible for people to buy Joy for All pets for use at home, and for innovative administrators at assisted living facilities to give the pets a try without breaking their budget. For example, Joy for All pets have been used successfully in the Memory Care wing at the Hebrew Home for the Aged in Riverdale, New York, in the Bronx, according to a report in the *New York Times,* as well as in Brookdale Communities around the country. They are also being tested in VA hospitals in California, among other places.

There is great deal of anecdotal support for these toy companions among family members who have witnessed their impact on their older relatives. For example, in "Letter of Recommendation: Hasbro Joy for All," an article published on March 24, 2016, in the *New York Times Magazine*, writer Jeremy D. Larson described a visit with his 91-year-old grandmother with dementia, who was living in a Memory Care facility in Florida. Larson noted that he had to introduce himself to his grandmother as her grandson when he walked into her room, and how difficult a relationship could be with someone who was drifting away. He wrote, "But when my grandmother ran her hand along Kitty's faux fur, and I saw that smile overtake her face, something changed . . . the grandmother I hadn't seen in years had arrived in order to care for the robot cat. Her happiness filled the room."

If you scan the reviews from online vendors, you can see the breadth and scope of the Joy for All Companion Pets' appeal. The majority of testimonials are from people who purchased a Companion Pet for an older relative, but there are reviews from other buyers as well. For example, there are parents who bought the pet for their autistic child, a boyfriend who had given one to his girlfriend who "loved it" and a mother who had bought one for her single adult daughter, but who ended up keeping it herself because her daughter was insulted that her mother thought she was lonely.

Given the popularity of the Companion Pet product line, it could be spun into a platform for creating new types of health products that bring "joy" into otherwise joyless activities for aging loved ones. As Fischer notes, "People don't want products that are too intrusive on their daily lives, but do crave products that help make daily, often unnecessary, tasks more enjoyable. Wouldn't it be great if a trusted Companion Pet could make mundane tasks more fun for older adults and their caregivers?" Fisher won't go into any details, but says the company is excited about the response to the Joy for All Companion Pet line and remains committed to "creating the world's best play experiences for people of all ages."

Bringing "joy" into the practice of medicine, as Fischer describes, may seem irrelevant in today's healthcare system, where the focus is on improving outcomes and efficiencies. But it could be as essential for health and wellness as any other therapy.

It's interesting to note that a chapter on "well-being" and aging has touched upon such a wide range of topics—medical and nonmedical—from hearing loss to loneliness, dementia, heart disease and the importance of purpose. But these seemingly disparate topics are all interconnected, just as our emotional state and our physical health are inextricably linked.

This brings me back to a subject I covered in Chapter 1—ageism. How people perceive aging and growing older appears to have a profound impact on their physical and mental health. I can think of no better way to end this chapter than to cite this insightful quote from Charlotte Yeh, *"If we can keep aging from becoming a state of boredom, uselessness and loneliness, we can literally change aging from a state to be feared to one we can embrace with anticipation and joy."*

◆ ◆ ◆

LAURA LANDRO: "THE "INFORMED PATIENT" ON THE PAST AND THE FUTURE

Laura Landro is a former *Wall Street Journal* editor and "The Informed Patient" columnist. She is author of *Survivor: Taking Control of Your Fight Against Cancer* (Simon & Schuster, 1998). In 1991, Landro was the media and marketing editor for the *Wall Street Journal* when, at age 37, she was diagnosed with chronic myelogenous leukemia, a potentially fatal blood cancer. Her book chronicles her journey from receiving a grim—and shocking—diagnosis to using her journalism skills to become an "expert" on her condition and ultimately undergoing a bone marrow transplant that saved her life.

Since 2002, Landro has been covering the healthcare system from the patient perspective. Below she shares some insights on healthcare then and now. I have known her for years and she represents everything that is right about journalism—she's professional, thoughtful and always seeking the truth. Her columns managed to catch the wave of what was on the mind of activated patients time and again.

Once you received your diagnosis, you dedicated yourself to learning as much as you could about your disease. How was your experience back in 1991 different than it would be today?

In 1991, there was no Google or simple way to access information. I was fortunate because, as an editor and reporter for the *Wall Street Journal*, I had access to medical studies through parent company Dow Jones's electronic news retrieval system and LEXIS/NEXIS. But it was nowhere as comprehensive as it is today. I was not able to easily access medical papers—the reality is, it's still tough to get ahold of medical research. Unfortunately, a lot of it is not open source or you can read the abstracts online but you can't get the actual papers. I think that needs to change.

Back then, there was no way to connect with other patients to understand what they had been through. Today you've got social media. In that respect, I think in many ways we're much luckier today. I had to ask my doctor to put me in touch with someone else who'd had a bone marrow transplant. I was able to talk to only one person who had had it; today, I would have been able to easily find other people to talk to online.

There are countless numbers of patient groups that have evolved from the original email listserv groups, like the Association of Cancer Online Resources (ACOR), started by Gilles Frydman in 1995. There are also tons of message boards and different Twitter groups and Facebook groups and really amazing disease advocacy groups. You can do all this research through your devices. There are so many groups, and so much to go through, I think it can be a bit overwhelming.

Speaking of overwhelming, over the past decade there has been an explosion in health apps and connected health tools. What needs to be done to make them useful to both consumers and healthcare professionals?

There are thousands of health apps and most of them don't have any real evidence behind them. We don't know that they are effective or that they help patients. But I think the most important thing for the medical profession to understand is that the only way it can really help patients with these digital tools is to be on the other end of them. There needs to be more information provided to the public, more monitoring of these tools. And people need to be kept informed of what's going on, either through text messaging or different forms of communication, so that they can stay on top of things. For example, it's not enough to give people an app to track their medications. Someone has to make sure that people are adhering to their medication schedule. And there needs to be a way of staying in touch with people, and not just when they're face-to-face with their healthcare team.

Even if you're a cancer patient, and you're going in for your infusions once a week or once every two weeks, how do you connect with a healthcare team in the times between that? What would be great is a tool that would really help people report their symptoms. There are some really interesting things going on now, like with COPD and remote sensors. A lot of this stuff is out there but you really have to prove that it's useful for patients, that patients can use it and feel that there's somebody on the other end who's paying attention to whatever data they're putting in or whatever questions they're asking.

Many people are fearful about having their medical information breached, but you have been very open about your issues.

Medical privacy is a personal, unique thing. I decided long ago to give up some of my medical privacy because I felt that after I went through all the stuff I did, as a journalist, I had to tell people about this so something good might come out of it—other than me living. At the *Wall Street Journal*, I wrote a travel column called "The Finicky Traveler" on the side for several years, and I felt that if it did nothing else, it empowered people to march up to the front desk and say, 'That room you've given me is no good, I'd like you to show me another one.'

Similarly, I felt that I could now tell people, 'Hey you can go to your doctor and challenge what they're saying, and you can do your own research and ask questions.'

You have to remember, when I first started doing this, it still was before the activated, engaged patient concept. It was 'doctor knows best,' and as a patient you just went to a doctor's appointment and they told you what to do. It was all still evolving.

How do we balance privacy concerns with the benefits of health technology?

As open as I have been about my condition, I don't want my health information being leaked. And obviously there are people who may have information that they don't want their insurance company to know. People are terrified of losing insurance coverage. And they're terrified their employer is going to discriminate against them, for example, if they have had cancer. These are all valid and legitimate concerns. People have sexually transmitted diseases or they have conditions that they don't want people to know about, to judge them. That's all completely understandable, but there's got to be a way to keep that information from being hacked or revealed and still deliver healthcare technology and improved health.

And there may be ways to compensate people for their information. Let's just say that you're a diabetic with a digital health app that's measuring your blood sugar and daily activity level, which could be really helpful to you. In exchange for wearing the device and allowing a third party access to your data, maybe you would see some pop-up ads on your phone saying, 'These are some products that people with diabetes like you find to be useful.' Is that worth it to you? Many people would say yes.

I'd like to add that people often forget how much privacy they have already given up quite willingly. I make every restaurant reservation, I do all my bill paying, I do all my banking, I do all my travel booking online, and I have given up enough information. I always say, why are we worried about the National Security Agency (NSA), when we've given all that information to Facebook and Google? They could hit you with a drone strike right now if they wanted to. That's my attitude about our concerns about privacy versus health.

How do you think technology will change how we age?

No one gets out of here alive, obviously! So you can extend life a certain amount, but the more you extend life and the older patients are, it's more likely they will be living with more chronic conditions and not managing them well. Many older people have multiple chronic conditions. For these people, I think that remote monitoring—especially remote monitoring to ensure medication adherence—could make a big difference. So can using other apps and tracking tools to monitor health right in the home.

As the baby boomer generation ages, obviously this is not a new thought. We're all used to our devices, so I think we need to really integrate that aging process with these devices. That way, you could live alone or be independent, but always know that there is technology available to either summon help or keep monitoring things you might not be aware of—like, oh my gosh, you don't know that your blood pressure's up or your cholesterol's soaring, or that you might be at risk for a pulmonary embolism or something. There are sensors that could be stuck on your body like an estrogen patch that would help detect those problems early, before they become life threatening. That, to me, would be the ideal for aging.

Medicare is exploring these options but we're still going to have to figure out how to fund it. Can we change this kind of fee-for-service healthcare system? It's gradually plodding toward quality; healthcare providers are getting paid for quality care, paid for outcomes, paid for being able to reduce hospitalizations and readmissions. So at what point does a model emerge that says we're going to pay for managing these digital applications and remote monitoring the same way we pay for an office visit?

What do you think is the most important trend right now in healthcare?

There's a lot going on, but I'm very interested in the work being done by the Patient-Centered Outcomes Research Institute (PCORI). The institute is funded through the Patient-Centered Outcomes Research Trust Fund (PCORTF), which was established by Congress through the Patient Protection and Affordable Care Act of 2010. It was founded to help doctors and patients work collaboratively to enable patients to make better-informed decisions and healthcare choices for themselves. In this model of shared decision making, patients and doctors evaluate the current research, weigh the pros and cons of different treatments and reach a decision together about how to proceed.

This is important because there is a lot of research that shows what's important to patients sometimes isn't what their doctors think it is. It goes into the end-of-life questions or the cancer treatment questions. At what point do you say, 'I don't want this quality of life that involves all these invasive medical treatments. I would like something less invasive that allows me to live my life, and maybe it won't be forever.' That to me is as interesting as anything is. When you actually get patients really involved in research and you ask them questions other than measuring what their symptoms are, you can begin to understand what they really want. And, as I said, it may not be what the doctor thinks they want.

This circles back to using technology to provide information. There's so much bad information out there, it is vital that patients have access to solid, well-vetted resources.

CHAPTER 8

The Art and Science of Caregiving

> *"Families come to us for help because a spouse has had a stroke or a cancer diagnosis, or a sibling has a severe mental disorder or other illness. Very often, they have children in the home. On top of that, they may also be caring for aging parents. Families are getting squeezed in every direction now, and it's just unbelievable."*
> —LINDSAY JURIST-ROSNER, CO-FOUNDER AND CEO, WELLTHY

> *"It doesn't matter how much you know and how prepared you are for it. When you're dealing with sick parents, it brings you to your knees."*
> —HEATHER M. YOUNG, PhD, RN, FAAN, FOUNDING DEAN, BETTY IRENE MOORE SCHOOL OF NURSING, UC DAVIS HEALTH

Today, 40 million Americans are providing assistance to an older parent, spouse or other loved one who is ill or needs care. *To put this figure in perspective, unpaid—and untrained—family members deliver around 80% of long-term care for aging relatives; one out of five families is involved in caregiving.* Although the responsibility of caring for older adults has traditionally fallen on their families, demographic and societal shifts over the past half-century are challenging caregivers in ways like never before:

- Thanks to advances in modern medicine, people are living longer, but at a price. Many are burdened with chronic diseases like diabetes, COPD, heart failure and cancer, requiring complex treatments and careful management.
- Most women—the traditional caregivers—are now employed outside the home. They are often juggling work, children and the needs of an older parent or spouse.
- Today, many family members often don't live in the same state—or country—as their loved ones and are forced to manage the care for an aging parent or parents from afar.

Caregiving can be very gratifying, but it can also exact a steep toll on the caregiver's emotional health and well-being. Studies show that assuming the role of caregiver puts you at higher risk for depression, heart disease, cancer and a slew of other ailments.

My father, who succumbed to Alzheimer's, lived with us for the last six months of his life. Although he never lost his dignity, caring for him was a tremendous amount of work for my wife and me. My youngest daughter grew very close to him during that phase and in some ways it was a joy to have him around. These are complex issues. As Lindsay Jurist-Rosner, co-founder and CEO of Wellthy, a startup providing family care coordination, notes, caregivers are being "squeezed in every direction." And it's going to get even worse.

Demographers call the year 2050, when the aging population will outnumber the younger population, "crossing the line." The primary concern among these experts is that there will be fewer working people to pay into Medicare and other programs to assist older adults. What isn't often discussed is that there will be too few humans—paid or unpaid—to care for the growing number of aging citizens.

We are beginning to feel the crunch right now. According to "Caregiving Innovation Frontiers," a 2016 study from AARP and Parks Associates, by 2020 an estimated 117 million Americans will need some form of assistance. This will further strain the resources of the projected 45 million available unpaid caregivers.

A 2016 study conducted by AARP on "Caregivers and Technology," found that 71% of the caregivers surveyed would be receptive to the idea of using technology to help provide care, but only around 7% actually use these tools. The report noted, "Barriers to technology adoption are wide and many, and caregivers perceive lack of awareness, cost, and time to find or learn about new technologies to be their greatest hurdles."

I refer once again to the nurse I described earlier in the book, who said that when he suggested to caregivers that they try out a new app or tool, their typical response was that they didn't want "one more thing to do." They didn't perceive of technology as making their lives easier, but as something that was only adding to their burden.

I submit that this is a failure of those of us who champion the use of technology in these situations. We've mostly designed our technologies to run in parallel with human interactions or, even worse, to supplant them. Virtually every service we consume other than healthcare has been made better by the thoughtful integration of technology to support human interactions (think Uber and Lyft). Conversely, in healthcare, we present technology that is viewed as "one more thing." This goes far beyond caregiving.

We need to do better: We need to create the right technologies that are simple and seamless, so that adoption is easy. And we need to work fast. Now more than ever, we need to be thinking about the ramifications of this demographic shift on the aging population. We need to be designing the tools that will lift the load for caregivers and enable older adults to better manage on their own. This chapter explores the coming "caregiver crisis" and how technology can improve the lives of both caregivers and the people who rely on them.

Having said this, I'd like to add two caveats: First, technology alone is not the sole solution to the problems facing caregivers, nor will it meet all the needs of those being "cared for." As the title of this chapter states, caregiving is very much an art—what I mean by that is that it needs to be done *artfully.* Technology needs to be respectful of both the feelings and privacy of the older adults who may need assistance. I noted earlier that people don't want to be spied on, or feel infantilized, or have their privacy violated, and I think that's something that tech developers often forget.

Second, there will never be a "one size fits all" plan for older adults. All older adults don't require the same kind or level of care. Some people will get by on little or no help other than a relative bringing food if it's snowy outside; others may require a more hands-on approach. Depending on the circumstance, the needs of an individual could change. That means we need to be flexible in our thinking.

Most of all, we have to start thinking and talking about this issue. Given the magnitude of this impending crisis, we hear surprisingly little about it. It is still very much a hidden problem. Perhaps our reluctance to discuss it is rooted in ageism. As individuals, we don't like to think about growing old or needing help with managing the tasks of everyday life.

And then there's the issue of money. As a society, we may be reluctant to offer more assistance to caregivers because of the potential cost. But we will pay dearly if we don't begin to tackle this problem before it blows up in our faces. If families are so overwhelmed that they can no longer function, and the needs of the elderly are neglected, it will result in more hospitalizations and nursing home admissions. That would not only be prohibitively expensive, but go against the wishes of an older population that wants to age in place and live as independently as possible.

Making the Healthcare System More Responsive

AARP has been working to raise awareness of the challenges confronting caregivers. As noted earlier, they have conducted several studies investigating the problems confronting this largely unrecognized workforce.

AARP has also been a strong advocate for the Caregiver Advise, Record, Enable (CARE) Act. The proposed law aims to provide better support, education and communication between hospitals and family caregivers as loved ones transition between hospital and home. The CARE Act requires hospitals to record the name of the family caregiver when the relative is admitted to the hospital, alert the family caregiver when the patient is discharged and provide basic education regarding the medical tasks the caregiver will be asked to perform when the patient gets home. As of this writing, it has been passed by 30 state legislatures.

It may seem obvious that medical professionals should keep family members in the loop—especially if they are the ones who will be assisting an older relative after a hospital stay—but that isn't always the case. According to Heather M. Young, founding dean of the Betty Irene Moore School of Nursing, part of UC Davis Health, caregivers are often overlooked and ignored by the healthcare system. "For the most part, our healthcare is set up on an individual care encounter; it's not based on a family model of thinking about caring for an individual," Young asserts. "There are a few exceptions, however," she notes. "For example, a pediatric nurse wouldn't do anything without involving the family, but that typically doesn't happen in geriatrics."

As Young observes, despite the fact that they are not always included in discussions related to the care plan, caregivers are taking on more responsibility than ever before. She notes that about half of the people who are discharged from the hospital will be asked to perform tasks at home that she would be reluctant to ask a first-year nursing student to perform without training. Yet, that's exactly what family caregivers are expected to do.

"They'll be told to change their relative's wound dressing when they get home, which is really scary," Young explains. "They'll be asked to manage their relative's ostomy bag. They have no training for it, no preparation and often have quite an emotional, negative reaction to doing it. They say, 'Oh, you've got to be kidding. I've got to do that for my mother or my father?'"

As Young says, the demands on caregivers are great, but support is often lacking. To fill this gap, the Betty Irene Moore School of Nursing is launching the Family Caregiving Institute to provide information, education, tools and services to this overworked, often unappreciated and fast-growing population. "We need to develop a better understanding of what families actually need, in terms of support from health systems. In particular, we need to focus on what competencies family members may need to develop, in order to enact their role as caregiver," Young explains.

Young adds that the Family Caregiving Institute will also work closely with healthcare professionals. "We need to help them get up to speed with this new paradigm because they weren't trained to work this way with families," she says.

The concept for the Family Caregiving Institute evolved from discussions on the future of healthcare between Young and Thomas S. Nesbitt, MD, MPH, associate vice chancellor for Strategic Technologies and Alliances at UC Davis Health. "Tom and I have been talking about how we get ahead of the shift from hospital-clinic-based care to providing care to where health actually happens—which is everywhere," Young says. "And we also have been looking for ways to support people as they age. We realized that it's not just about helping people manage health in an episodic fashion—for example, after they've had a fall and broken a hip. We needed to provide a way for people to plan and manage their health over a long period of time."

According to Nesbitt, the Family Caregiving Institute is looking to develop a wide range of technologies to assist caregivers, either in partnership with other companies or tapping into the vast resources of UC Davis. Nesbitt notes that the team is focusing on three different areas where technology could be useful: "First, there are technologies for the 'body,' which include biometric trackers that measure things like blood pressure, heart rate and blood sugar levels," Nesbitt explains. "Second, there are the technologies for the 'home,' like embedded sensors or smart TVs, which can be used to store medical information and video conferencing. Third, there are the technologies for 'community interaction,' which enable caregivers and older adults to connect with others for support and information sharing."

And down the road, Nesbitt also sees a role for robotics.

"Heather [Young] talks about the need for 'brawn and brain' in technology," Nesbitt says. "We are hoping to develop robotic technology that can provide assistance with tasks such as transfers from bed to a wheelchair—that's the brawn part. At the same time, we're exploring using machine learning so that the robot can predict when someone wants to get up before they start to do it by themselves and fall down. That's the 'brain' part. We need to make this technology as simple for users as possible, so that they don't have to figure out how to call the robot to help them; the robot knows what to do."

The Family Caregiving Institute aims to be a hub of information for caregivers, providing access to evidence-based information and tools, to instill both competency and confidence. For example, even before the formal launch of the institute, the Betty Irene Moore School of Nursing at UC Davis had partnered with both AARP and the Home Alone Alliance to create videos for people who are being discharged from hospitals, to enable them or their caregivers to perform the necessary follow-up at home.

Young explains, "We've done a series on medication, explaining topics such as how to give injections and administer eye drops. We did a series on mobility, which included how you get in and out of a car with a wheelchair and how to go up stairs with a walker. And we just did a series on wound care—we covered how to manage those really complicated, nasty wounds."

The instructional videos are not only intended to educate people, but also to provide emotional support for those who may be feeling uneasy about their new role. As Young says, "The videos are not just about 'how to do' things. We also say, 'Yeah, we understand this is really scary and we have some suggestions on how to help you better manage all of this.'"

When it comes to technology, the UC Davis team understands that people cannot be expected to readily accept costly and complicated new gadgets into their home. So they are working on repurposing technologies that are already in the home, to enable people to live independently in a safer environment.

For example, Nesbitt says a home security system can be programmed to alert a remote caregiver to whether an older relative has opened the refrigerator door or bathroom door by a certain time during the day, which would indicate that they are mobile and taking care of the activities of daily living. Or a smart TV can be programmed to remind people to take their medication. It can also be used for video chats with doctors or nurses, or even as a way to deliver physical therapy into the home, a project that they are already working on with Microsoft technology.

"Our researchers have repurposed the Xbox One Kinect gaming system for creating gamification of rehabilitation exercises. The idea would be that if you do your rotator cuff exercise correctly, you would get points for it," Nesbitt explains. The next step is to program the system to automatically send the information to the patient's physical therapist for review, as well as incorporate the data into the user's medical record. There have been a number of efforts over the years to do remote physical therapy and the technology piece is often just a bit too difficult or expensive to deal with. This is an important area for innovation and we're on the cusp of getting it right.

Young and Nesbitt have laid out an ambitious agenda, and Nesbitt says that it will take about a decade to fully develop the Family Caregiving Institute. This is important work. Efforts such as this will add to our collective knowledge of how best to solve this vexing problem of caring for people when those who need care outnumber those who can give it. One of the most important things to watch is going to be what the right mix of technology will be and how it will complement the human interactions.

On the Frontline: A Caregiver's Startup

Caregiving for an older adult can be a complex undertaking that requires a great deal of multitasking. In some cases, you not only have the responsibility of making sure that your loved one is following a medication protocol or doing his physical therapy or even eating regular meals, but you may also be managing a paid caregiver. It can get very time-consuming and complicated.

People who can afford it can seek the services of a geriatric care manager to help design a plan, or hire prescreened home aides. Even so, the day-to-day part of management often falls to the family caregiver. There are a number of new startups trying to fill this need, including the following:

- *Honor.* Founded in 2015, the company promises to deliver "home care your family will love." Honor links family members to prescreened, paid caregivers who work in the home. As part of its service, the company offers an app for family members to stay in touch with the caregiver. As of this writing, Honor provides services in select cities in California, Texas and New Mexico.

- *Hometeam.* Founded in 2013 by Josh Bruno, a former investor at Bain Ventures, Hometeam places in-home, paid caregivers throughout New York, New Jersey and Pennsylvania. The service offers an iPad app that sends daily emails to family caregivers so they can keep track of what's going with their relative, and immediately alerts them if there's a problem.

- *CareLinx.* Founded in 2011, CareLinx is one of the most established of these startups. The company operates nationwide, matching people to the right caregiver, as well as offering an app that enables the family to text and talk to the caregiver in real time. The company claims that the virtual caregiving agency is saving consumers up to 50% over what it would cost to work with a brick-and-mortar agency. In 2012, CareLinx was the winner of AARP's Consumer Award, announced at their Health Innovation@50+ Live Pitch, held in New Orleans.

There are other similar companies popping up around the country and, given the dire circumstances facing many caregivers, these services are filling an important need. Undoubtedly, we will see even more companies like these in the not-too-distant future.

One startup in particular, Wellthy, captured our imagination because of the personal story and vision of its co-founder, Lindsay Jurist-Rosner.

In Chapter 2, Michael Greeley of Flare Capital noted that investors are now beginning to look at companies that provide "comprehensive services for family caregivers," like screening of for-hire caregivers, meal delivery and automated prescription renewal, as well as tools linking them to prescreened caregivers. In other words, they're interested in companies that provide "one-stop shopping" for overwhelmed and overstretched caregivers. That's exactly what Lindsay Jurist-Rosner had in mind when she founded Wellthy.

Jurist-Rosner understood the strains that were being placed on caregivers because, for most of her life, she has been one. When she was 9 years old, her mother was diagnosed with advanced primary progressive multiple sclerosis, a degenerative disease of the central nervous system. At an early age, Jurist-Rosner learned what it meant to be a caregiver, navigating the healthcare system while balancing her school and work life to help her mother out as much as she could.

In her mid-20s, Jurist-Rosner took a job in digital marketing for a California tech company, 3,000 miles away from her mother in Washington, DC. On many weekends, she found herself taking the red eye back to DC to deal with medical and other crises related to her mother's condition. Exhausted and overwhelmed by her experience, Jurist-Rosner decided to use her tech skills to "bring caregiving into the twenty-first century." In December 2014, she and Goldman Sachs alum Kevin Roche co-founded Wellthy, a startup providing support to families with complex care needs.

Jurist-Rosner, who earned a BA in Economics-Operations Research from Columbia and an MBA from Harvard, is a former ad tech executive for digital and media companies. Roche graduated with a BS in Computer Science and Math from Northeastern University.

Wellthy is a care concierge, helping manage healthcare for families with sick and aging loved ones. Families get a dedicated care coordinator (think personal healthcare assistant) who creates a plan and gets tasks done, all through a modern online experience. Tasks include: scheduling appointments, refilling prescriptions, handling prior authorizations, sourcing and vetting the right in-home aide, handling a move into a care facility, contesting insurance bills and much more.

Simply put, Wellthy does indeed offer the one-stop shopping Michael Greeley describes above and is an invaluable partner for families, providing expertise and getting things done across a wide range of medical, social and financial issues. Prospective clients can sign up on Wellthy.com, or by calling a toll-free number. The family is then matched to a care coordinator, one of the hundreds of social workers around the United States who work as independent contractors for the startup. After asking the prospective clients questions, either by phone or over the proprietary messaging platform, the care coordinator designs what Jurist-Rosner describes as a "digital game plan."

Jurist-Rosner says that when people contact Wellthy they are usually at the end of their rope, overwhelmed by all the basic things that need to get done for the person that they're caring for. For starters, they may have to deal with finances, insurance companies, medication prescriptions, a pile of hospital bills—and that's just the tip of the iceberg. If the person wants to remain in his or her home, the family has to help make all of those arrangements too.

Jurist-Rosner explains, "The care coordinator acts like a project manager, helping prioritize: 'First things first, we're going to tackle this piece right now because we need to figure this piece out before we can figure out this piece and this piece.' And then they just get to work."

Private clients are charged $300 a month to work with a care coordinator; $200 a month if they commit to six months in advance. Wellthy is also selling its services to employers and Jurist-Rosner says they have been very receptive. "We've started talking to some benefits leaders at top companies. And as we explain what we are doing and what we are solving for—a parent with dementia, a spouse with cancer, a child with special needs, a sibling with a mental health situation—the benefits leaders' heads start nodding, often admitting this is a huge gap in their current offering."

Since its founding, Wellthy has devoted a great deal of time and resources to building a proprietary platform from the ground up, which Jurist-Rosner describes as a "modern and seamless" experience for families. "We provide a secure online account for the family, where every piece of information pertaining to the 'care project' is stored and tracked in their account," she explains. "The online account has the digital care plan; private, secure and encrypted document storage, which families use to capture legal documents, like a power of attorney or living will, and medical records; and medication and contact trackers."

According to Jurist-Rosner, the most powerful feature of the Wellthy platform is its "multi-stakeholder communication." It allows all family members who want to be involved in the care project to easily follow along and receive updates from the care coordinator simultaneously, regardless of where they may be living. It is a boon for people who are trying to manage care for a relative who may live far away.

The shared platform also enables care coordinators to learn from one another, creating a rich database of family caregiving experiences that can be tapped to streamline and improve the caregiving process. "We see everything that the healthcare system doesn't see," Jurist-Rosner says. "The healthcare system only sees what happens in clinical settings, and family caregiving takes place outside of traditional healthcare settings. We're able to capture all of the nonclinical data. This allows us to learn from these situations, so that with every family we work with, we get better, and we're able to service families more cost efficiently due to this central knowledge base. It's sort of like crowdsourcing among the care coordinators that we've built into the platform."

Jurist-Rosner understands the power of data and how it can be used to transform both the caregiver experience and the healthcare system itself. She notes that, as the technology gets smarter, Wellthy will be able to incorporate more automation and machine learning into its program. The goal is to enable the company to move from crisis intervention to predictive analytics.

"Eventually, we will be able to predict what families need before they even know that they need it," Jurist-Rosner says. "The other real goal of the data, for me, is how do we use the data we're collecting to improve care and improve health, and improve the country, right, improve healthcare costs? I don't know what the answer is to these questions, but I feel strongly that over the next five years, we'll start to get there."

Wellthy is still relatively small; only several thousand people are enrolled for its services. However, it is in the process of signing up several companies that will offer the service to their employees, and that will extend their coverage to the tens of thousands. In 2016, the company raised $2 million in seed money, much of it devoted to developing its technology. The company is now moving to a Series A round of funding in the second half of 2017.

Companies that provide eldercare coordination are bound to take off as the population ages and more and more grown children find themselves responsible for the safety and well-being of their parents, spouses and other loved ones.

A Robot in Every Home?

Most of us have the best of intentions when it comes to helping out older relatives and friends who need us, but it's not always possible to meet all of their needs. For one thing, as I mentioned earlier, we may find ourselves living and working thousands of miles away from our loved ones. For another, as the older population increases and the younger population shrinks, younger relatives and friends may be caring for more people than they can humanly manage. Even if they have the money to pay for help—and many people don't—there may be a shortage of paid caregivers, which will drive the cost up even further. That leaves us no choice but to develop some nonhuman options.

When it comes to preparing for the future of its aging population, by necessity, Japan is well ahead of the rest of the world in developing humanoid robots. Today, more than 25% of Japan's population is over 65 and that will grow to 40% by 2050. That country is already feeling the pinch of too few people to care for too many. In 2015, the Japanese government outlined "Japan's Robot Strategy," a five-year plan launched by its Ministry of Economy, Trade and Industry to spark robot innovation, which included creating robots to assist in nursing homes and hospitals, and as companions for older adults.

Long before its official "robot strategy," Japan was in the vanguard of robots. Back in 2000, Tokyo-based Honda introduced Japan's most famous robot, ASIMO, which stands for Advanced Step in Innovative Mobility. ASIMO is billed as the most advanced humanoid robot in the world. Upgraded in 2011, ASIMO has had its ups and downs, including a few bungled demos. At well over $1 million or so per unit, it has been dismissed as an "overpriced toy," but that's selling it—and robotics—short.

At 4'3" and 119 pounds, ASIMO looks a bit like a clunky storm trooper right out of a *Star Wars* movie, but it has some impressive capabilities. Click onto its website and you will see ASIMO strut its stuff— walking, climbing steps and dancing around with relative ease. Honda boasts that ASIMO recognizes objects, gestures and the environment.

What's most impressive is a YouTube video showing ASIMO pushing a medicine cart and using its five-fingered mechanical hands to carefully pour a drink out of a container into a glass without spilling a drop. Sure, it's still a bit slow on task, but it doesn't take a great leap of imagination to see that ASIMO, or robots like it, will one day be bopping down the corridors of a hospital or nursing home. The price will have to come down significantly before ASIMO or other robots will be mainstreamed. But given the history of tech, it's a good bet that it will eventually happen.

There are other "celebrity" robots in Japan, including Pepper, a more affordable device manufactured by Softbank and Aldebaran Robotics, which retails for around $1,700 and comes with additional monthly fees. Given its petite size, Pepper is not designed for heavy lifting, but with its perky personality it is being touted as an ideal companion for older adults.

It's got commercial applications too: Versions of it are being used in retail spaces to engage customers. Pepper communicates through speech and an interactive screen embedded on its child-sized body, which is perched on top of a three-wheel omnidirectional base. It has humanlike arms and hands and a moveable head. Its big eyes are equipped with 3-D cameras that can detect people and its surroundings, and decode facial expressions. And it talks and sings in a cute, childlike voice. (My co-author Carol encountered a Pepper at a shop in Narita Airport in Tokyo last year and was regaled with the robot's version of the Macarena.) Pepper is already being tested in nursing homes in Japan and can be purchased from the company for home and commercial use.

There are also home robots on the US market right now: Amazon's Alexa and Google Home are personal home assistants that function in the social robot category. In Chapter 5, I wrote about Mabu, a social robot being developed to help people better manage their chronic illnesses. And while we don't yet have robots as advanced as Rosie, the iconic maid on the *Jetsons* who could cook, clean and manage the kids, there are some interesting home robots on the horizon that can help fill the caregiver gap.

One of them is made by OhmniLabs, a Santa Clara, California–based robotics startup from StartX, a nonprofit accelerator program funded by Stanford University and others. OhmniLabs recently launched its own home telepresence family robot. The basic structure is a tablet enabled with two-way video chat capability on a pole connected to a moveable three-wheel base. The robot (Ohmni) can be controlled remotely by authorized users across town—or halfway across the world. As the older adult chats with a relative and moves around her home, the robot moves with her. As OhmniLab's website notes, Ohmni enables users to "cook together, watch a video or attend a family dinner or a loved one's birthday party."

The desire to stay in touch with family was the driving force behind the creation of OhmniLabs, which was founded in 2015 by serial entrepreneurs Thuc Vu, Tingxi Tan and Jared Go. Vietnam-born Vu, who has a PhD in computer science from Stanford University, had worked as a computer engineer for Google and already had several successful startups under his belt. Vu and Go met when they were undergraduates at Carnegie Mellon University and reunited at Stanford, where they started brainstorming about founding a company together.

They decided whatever it turned out to be, their company had to be meaningful and fill a need. Both Vu and Go had families back in Vietnam, whom they were rarely able to see. And that distance gave them an idea. They knew that telepresence robots were big in business and industry, but had not caught on in the home. So they decided to build a robot that could enable families to share experiences with each other, even if they could no longer spend face-to-face time together.

"Even though I try to go home as often as I can, my parents and my grandma live in Vietnam. That's 21 hours of flying and traveling time to get there," Vu explains. "We wanted to make a product that allows us to be home instantly to see our families. And it wasn't just for our benefit. When we developed the robot and tested it in front of people, we found that there's a huge value that we can provide to the senior population."

Vu notes that one of Ohmni's missions is to combat loneliness and isolation, a major problem among the elderly, especially those who feel left behind after family members have moved away. Some people were skeptical as to whether or not older people would accept a robot into their homes. But the desire to interact with family quickly dissolved any initial discomfort with robots. As Vu says, "Sure, first the usual response is 'Hmm this is kind of weird. I'm not sure if I'm comfortable with this.' Then when their family members pop up on the screen and start talking, all their reservations just go out the window. The seniors love it."

OhmniLabs went to great lengths to build a robot that is easy to use. The robot arrives fully assembled, with instructions to just "unbox, unfold and connect to Wi-Fi." There is no software to upload and no learning curve for the primary user. The robot is the size of a small human—4'8"—with a movable neck that can tilt forward and nod in agreement. It has an integrated screen. The robot's actions are controlled by the remote user, who can also charge the robot by using a built-in auto-docking feature. (The robot can run for about five hours between charges.) Ohmni weighs 18 pounds, only slightly more than many home vacuum cleaners, and folds in half so that it can be moved around easily. Any authorized user with access to the Internet can join the conversation.

Unlike a Skype call or FaceTime on a smartphone or conventional tablet, Ohmni can follow someone around his or her home, so a conversation can occur in a more natural manner. "One of my favorite uses is to learn how to cook family recipes from my grandma. I have the robot in my family home in Vietnam and just dial it in and follow my grandmother into the kitchen and learn how to cook from her. Because everything is operated remotely, seniors can continue to do what they are doing. For them, it is a totally hands-free experience. They don't need to handle or hold onto a tablet or a computer as in Skype. They can continue knitting, cooking or watching television. I can join in that experience with them and share those moments with them."

OhmniLabs has piloted Ohmni at The Heritage Downtown senior living apartments in Walnut Creek, California, where, according to Jenny Shively, resident relations director, it's been a big hit. Two residents are using Ohmni in their apartments and a third unit is placed in the lobby for all residents to use. "It attracts a great deal of attention," Shively says. "Our residents love the robot. They are not the least bit intimidated by it. They're not shy about getting it exactly the way they want."

A New Model for Caregiving

Vu notes that Ohmni is not just a way for families to visit together, but enables remote caregivers to keep an eye on a loved one in a friendly, nonintrusive way. For example, while you are moving around the home with a relative, you can get a good idea of his or her living conditions, physical state and cognitive function. But Vu cautions against "spying," and notes that although the robot is always connected, when the older adult doesn't want "company," she can turn off the screen whenever she feels like it. That way, if someone dials in, she doesn't have to accept the call.

Vu adds that it is essential for tech developers to include these kinds of features, because older people in particularly want to maintain both their dignity and privacy. "We need to be sensitive about their need for privacy—it is even more important to them than to the younger generation. They don't want to be made to feel weak or dependent. And they don't want to feel like they're being watched all the time. That's why many of them hate security cameras in the home and don't want to use wearables."

Right now, Ohmni is still a sophisticated communications tool, but Vu has a much bigger vision for his robot. OhmniLabs is inviting businesses and developers to build custom integrations onto its platform.

Vu believes that Ohmni will become the hub of the Internet of Healthy Things tech in the home. "In fact because of the way we designed the robot, it's very easy to add on medical devices like wearables, which can send data back to the robot," he says. "This way, from a remote location, the caregiver can walk the senior through measuring blood pressure and heart rate, and then transfer that information to the doctor. And doctors can call in remotely as well, in case the senior has some issues or questions. That will be the next step after we get into the home and provide the basic service."

Vu also predicts that future generations of Ohmni will be able to perform tasks in the home, like lifting objects or assisting people in and out of a chair.

Down the road, Vu says that Ohmni can provide a new model of caregiving; one in which a centrally located caregiver can check in on several older adults remotely, without having to do it in person. "From a remote location, a caregiver can make sure that people are taking their medications properly, are following their diets, and remind them of their doctor's appointments, those kinds of basic things," Vu says. He adds that if someone needs hands-on help for things like bathing or cooking, a caregiver can come over to help the person perform those specific tasks, but doesn't have to be there all the time.

In April 2017, OhmniLabs launched Ohmni in an Indiegogo campaign that offered the robot to subscribers for $1,395, nearly a third less than its projected retail price. The campaign exceeded expectations and production is gearing up for more units. Vu says that every unit is built at the OhmniLabs' Santa Clara headquarters; he estimates that the company will soon be able to turn out about 1,000 units annually.

We're Still on the Ground Floor

There's a great deal more work to be done to relieve the burden on caregivers and enable those in their care to live safely and as independently as possible in their homes. It's a very positive sign that startups are venturing into this space, and while many of these companies offer services that are helpful, no one has gotten it completely right yet. Caregiving is still too difficult and too fragmented.

The bottom line is, no one has applied seamless, simple "Uber-like" design to this space—an app that coordinates everything for both the caregiver and older adult. The field is ripe for more innovation. I am posing a challenge to entrepreneurs and developers: Do better. Think about all the tools that have made your life easier—from online banking to food delivery services and digital health trackers—and try to adapt them for caregivers.

For starters, here are some features that I would like to see integrated within one app, which can be used by both the caregiver and older adult:

- Passive, in-home monitoring of an older adult (that doesn't infringe upon his privacy), which enables the caregiver to make sure that the person is up and moving around. This can be done using embedded sensors placed strategically around the home or via the GPS in a smart device.
- Automated medication adherence monitoring that doesn't rely on an elder's self-reporting, as well as automatic reordering of prescriptions.
- Vital sign monitoring, as appropriate, to the level of the condition.
- The use of vocal analytics and/or face decoding technology to detect subtle but early changes in cognition, health and mood, as described in Chapter 5.
- Easy and effortless connectivity for both the elder and the caregiver and back, as well as to the medical team, social services, payers and all other appropriate parties.
- Automatic alerts sent to a caregivers and their charge's family, both to assure them when the elder is doing well and to alert them when the elder is not.
- Integration with a car service like Circulation (described in Chapter 2).
- Integration with a grocery and/or meal delivery service.

Much of this could run on Amazon's Echo, Google Home or a similar platform. Some home care companies already offer some of these features, but to date no one offers the entire package. I predict that the company that comes up with a workable model will be very successful.

◆ ◆ ◆

NOT TOO HUMAN

"We anthropomorphize our pets; we anthropomorphize our cars and several tools and appliances around the house; so it's not that robots have to be human in order for us to initiate the script of a human-human communication. In fact, if they're too human that's when, actually, we might find it problematic, evoking this eerie, kind of creepy feeling, because they're trying to be something that they are not supposed to be."

—S. Shyam Sundar, PhD, distinguished professor and founding director of the Media Effects Research Lab at Penn State University's College of Communications

The thought of having robots as assistants or caregivers for older adults may seem a bit like science fiction. And it raises the questions: Just how comfortable will humans be living side by side with machines? Can we bond with nonliving "things"?

The answer is yes. In fact, we do it all the time. We humans can grow very attached to inanimate objects: The dolls, Furbys and stuffed animals that we played with during childhood seemed very real to us at the time. Adults also can develop "relationships" with inanimate objects. I've talked before about the "romance" between humans and their smartphones, and more than a few grown-ups have been known to grow so fond of their cars' navigation systems that they assign them a name. There is compelling evidence that people can form a bond with a virtual presence that is every bit as powerful as a human relationship.

At Partners Connected Health, we have explored different ways of using "relational agents," computer-generated avatars designed to bond with human beings and create relationships with people to encourage and motivate better self-care. I know that there are individuals who cling to the notion that people would never accept healthcare from virtual or robotic entities (which studies show is simply not true). But even if this was true, it's no longer feasible. Once you accept the fact that we are running out of human providers and caregivers to monitor people in a meaningful way, the only options left are robotic and/or virtual. Furthermore, the kinds of chronic health problems that people suffer from today require in-the-moment, real-time interventions that can keep people on track.

Many people need to be reminded when it's time to take their medication; they need support if they are feeling lonely or isolated. Some may need to be reminded to eat at mealtime or to do their physical therapy exercises every day. If they're not sleeping well at night, they need "someone" to talk to. It's impossible for even the most attentive provider or relative to be present at the precise moments, 24/7, when they are needed. Virtual caregivers and social robots have no lives of their own; they can be at our beck and call; they don't eat, sleep or take vacations.

Early in our research at Partners Connected Health, we were interested in seeing how people would react to working with an avatar. In one study, we collaborated with Tim Bickmore, PhD, professor at the College of Computer and Information Science at Northeastern University, to see how patients responded to a virtual health coach. Our goal was to improve walking behavior among sedentary patients. In our study, Karen, the virtual coach, simulated face-to-face conversation, including goal setting, positive reinforcement and education. The study showed that there was a significant increase in step count among the patients who had access to Karen, as opposed to those who were simply asked to walk more but did not have the additional virtual coach.

Other studies conducted by Bickmore's group have shown that many people actually prefer working with a virtual entity as opposed to a human being when receiving their discharge instructions from a hospital. Why? Patients reported that the avatar was a lot more patient than the human nurse, and it didn't talk down to them or make them feel embarrassed to ask the same question multiple times. So it's not a stretch to believe that given the opportunity, people would be willing to work with an avatar to help them better manage complicated health issues.

But how will people respond to robots—not just images on a screen, but life-size, if not lifelike, objects that exist side by side with us in the real world?

S. Shyam Sundar, PhD, is distinguished professor and founding director of the Media Effects Research Lab at Penn State University's College of Communications. Sundar investigates the "social and psychological effects of technological elements unique to online communication, ranging from websites to newer social media." And that includes human-social robot interactions. If social robots are going to be used to assist elderly people in a variety of tasks, it's important to know what people like and respond to, and what they find "creepy." In a study published in the January 2017 issue of the *International Journal of Human Computer Studies*, "Cheery Companions or Serious Assistants? Role and Demeanor Congruity as Predictors of Robot Attraction and Use intentions Among Senior Citizens," Sundar and his team reveal some fascinating insights.

The researchers recruited 51 residents of a senior living home in central Pennsylvania. The participants were given a smartphone and told that they could invite a robot to approach them. The robot was about 4' tall and equipped with a robotic arm, web camera and screen. The experiments involved four different scenarios: The robot was identified as either a companion robot or an assistant robot. The assistant robot was given either a serious or a playful demeanor, and the companion robot was also given either a serious or a playful demeanor. The purpose of the study was to see which type of robot the participants preferred for which task.

At first glance, the results were surprising, as Sundar explains. "The seniors actually liked a companion robot that was serious more than a companion robot that was playful, and when we dug into the reasons, the data showed that a companion robot that was playful was seen as being too eerily similar to a human," he says. "This is a phenomenon called uncanny valley. The robot would try to do some things that are almost human, and even though consciously people know it's not human, that's when it results in this feeling of uneasiness, eeriness and creepiness, if you will."

And just the opposite was true for the assistant robot, Sundar reports. "On the other hand, we found that it was desirable for an assistant robot to be playful rather than serious. In general, of course, assistant robots compared to companion robots elicit less-positive attitudes overall with seniors. They are less socially attractive for senior citizens, but the less-positive attitudes are somewhat diminished by the cheerfulness of the robot's personality."

My take on this is that an assistant robot that is serious may be too similar to an overly efficient home aide or family caregiver who is constantly reminding the elder of what he or she can no longer do. But if the assistant robot appears to be friendly and "playful," it may take the sting out of the fact that the individual needs assistance. As Sundar points out, we need to be sensitive to these issues before we fill up senior centers and nursing homes with social robots that we think people will like.

"These are the kinds of nuances that we should be thinking about and paying attention to when we try to design robots. The overwhelming model, for engineers at least, is to imitate human-human interaction in technology design," Sundar observes. "While a lot of social rules of human-human interaction are, in fact, replicated with human-computer interaction and sometimes human-robot interaction, there are certain aspects of humanness that we tend to get freaked out about. If 'it' imitates humanlike qualities, then we place a distance between us and 'it' because we are psychologically scared of it. Eerie is the best word for it."

So in the end, the robot that elicits the best emotional response from humans may be the one that's not "too human" and leaves a bit to the imagination. "On the other hand," Sundar notes, "if it's left to us, even if it's not particularly human-looking or not particularly humanlike, our default tendency is to treat it as human because of the built-in social script in our head that is automatically invoked whenever we interact."

CHAPTER 9

Cracking the Code for Healthy Longevity

"In many ways, our study is an aging study. We're going to study the life process of people of a whole different set of ages, and then follow them through end of life to understand what mattered and what didn't."
—Eric Dishman, director, the All of Us Research Program, National Institutes of Health

"We need to design early warning systems that identify that first transition from wellness to predisease, rather than waiting for a problem to actually reach the point where somebody is complaining of symptoms. That, I think, is a very different way of looking at biology. You're not saying, 'I'm going to define the disease in terms of a series of things that somebody complains about that lead to a general set of outcomes.' What you're saying is, 'I'm going to try and understand very specific biological processes before they ever really emerge as symptoms and then understand how to head them off at the pass.'"
—Calum MacRae, MD, PhD, head, the One Brave Idea research project, and chief of Cardiovascular Medicine at Brigham and Women's Hospital, Boston

f, by the turn of the next century, we have cracked the code on how to extend both lifespan and healthspan, it will be in large part due to the work being done today by medical researchers and scientists who are studying human life in ways that were never before possible.

Using new twenty-first century tools, like genomic sequencing, biometric sensors, electronic health records and even social media, these researchers are studying the interaction between *genotype*—your genes—and *phenotype,* an organism's observable characteristics or traits that are determined by genotype as well as by environmental influences. These two inputs are often referred to as "nature" and "nurture." Phenotype is a vast category that encompasses characteristics such as height and hair color, as well as biochemical or physiological properties, behavior, overall health and general disposition. Due to the influence of environmental factors, even people with identical genotypes, such as identical twins, can have nonidentical phenotypes.

Variations in phenotype could explain why people with similar genetics don't always develop the same diseases. It's why only some people with a gene that increases the risk of developing Alzheimer's disease, for example, will actually develop the disease but others won't. And it's why only some people with a strong family history for heart disease will actually develop heart problems. Ultimately, it could unravel the mystery as to why some people age better than others; why some people can run marathons at age 80 and others the same age can't take a step without a walker. It is the piece of the puzzle that has confounded physicians and researchers from time immemorial. And until it is solved, it is very difficult to provide insightful, personalized medicine targeted to the needs of each individual.

If this work pans out, it will provide a treasure trove of information about the onset of the chronic illnesses that have become a worldwide epidemic. And, more importantly, provide insights on how to identify these illnesses early in life when intervention is the most powerful, or perhaps even prevent them altogether.

In this final chapter, I highlight two extraordinary projects. First, the *All of Us* Research Program funded by the National Institutes of Health and headed by Eric Dishman. Second, One Brave Idea, a project co-funded by the American Heart Association (AHA), Google's Verily (formerly Google Life Sciences) and AstraZeneca, which is headed by Calum MacRae, MD, PhD, at Brigham and Women's Hospital in Boston.

These projects are big, bold and vast in scope. They are trailblazers in how they have been conceived and are being conducted, and even in their early stages, it's safe to say that they both have enormous potential to transform not only how future research projects are done, but the practice of medicine itself.

A Million Subjects

The *All of Us* Research Program, formerly known as the Precision Medicine Initiative Cohort Program, is a landmark, longitudinal study with the goal of enrolling *1 million Americans*. The study will track the lifestyle, behavior, medical history, biosamples (like blood and urine) and genomics over the lifespan of volunteers of all ages, from all ethnicities, in all stages of health and from all walks of life. This information will be linked to the electronic medical records of the participants. In the words of NIH Director Francis S. Collins, MD, PhD, it is an "audacious" study.

As stated on the *All of Us* website, its mission "is to accelerate health research and medical breakthroughs, enabling individualized prevention, treatment, and care for all of us." It promises to be a "highly interactive research model, with participants as partners in the development and implementation of the research and with significant representation in program governance and oversight."

Project director Dishman was an Intel Fellow who founded Intel's first Health Research and Innovation Lab in 1999 and Intel's Digital

Health Program in 2005. He is internationally acclaimed for spearheading research projects on technology, aging and independent living, which have been implemented worldwide. I've known Eric for many years and he has always been at the forefront of how technology will impact healthcare. His own bout with and victory over kidney cancer (as detailed below) has been, in large part, the inspiration for his efforts to transform healthcare.

Dishman understands from firsthand experience why this is such an important, potentially lifesaving endeavor. When he was a 19-year-old college sophomore, he was diagnosed with a rare form of kidney cancer. Told that there was no treatment or cure, he wasn't expected to survive more than a few years. For more than two decades, he was subjected to 62 rounds of chemotherapy and horrific side effects from medication. Finally, in his early 40s, it seemed as if he had reached the end of the road when his treatment options ran out. This story would have had a very different ending had he not bumped into a friend working at a DNA sequencing company: He suggested that Dishman have a whole genome sequence of his cancer cells. That led to a better understanding of Dishman's atypical form of cancer, a new and better-targeted treatment strategy and, ultimately, a cure.

Eric Dishman is well aware that he was extremely lucky to be in a position where he had access to the latest science, and he acknowledges that without it, he probably wouldn't be here today. His goal is to make the same cutting-edge, high-quality "precision medicine" that saved his life available to the rest of the population, and not just for cancer but for all diseases.

"The essence of precision medicine is finding the right tool for the job, for this person presenting at this time, given a wide range of data points about them," Dishman explains. "Do they need a drug? Do they need counseling? Do they need a coach? Do they need an app? It's about having a wider array of tools at our disposal, and only using the big, expensive tools like hospitals and expensive drugs when (a) we are absolutely certain that they're needed, and (b) we know that they're going to work for that particular individual."

Dishman believes that ultimately *All of Us* will help develop this "precision" model of a highly specific, personalized form of medicine targeted to the individual. But it won't happen overnight.

All of Us is a massive undertaking that involves many complex moving parts: Dishman estimates that it will take at least three to four years to fully implement the project. Once a million people are signed up, the amount of data that will be collected as part of this study is mind-boggling. "We believe this will be the largest biomedical data set in the world by far, because we are combing imaging, genomics, EHR, streaming data from wearables and all that. We will have some of the biggest computational and storage challenges of anybody," he says.

In June 2017, *All of Us* began enrolling its first participants as beta testers, an initial phase that launched the study with around10,000 research subjects. NIH is working with a team of universities, medical centers and technology companies that will help enroll participants and collect the bio-samples. Individuals are also invited to sign up on their own, either on *joinallofus.org* or through their healthcare providers. The study investigators will be doing frequent bio-sample collections, following up every 18 to 24 months.

At this stage, the study will not be collecting data from wearables. According to Dishman, that part of the study will be phased in sometime in 2018. The genomics part will be phased in later too.

Much has yet to be decided. For example, Dishman notes that his team has not selected the wearable or wearables that will be included in the study. The program is coordinating that effort with the Scripps

Transitional Science Institute, led by Eric Topol, MD. Dishman notes that they may begin by having people who are already using wearables share their data. Eventually NIH may design their own wearable or commission a tech company to develop a wearable device specific to the parameters that they want to study longitudinally.

That's a lot trickier than it sounds. Dishman explains, "Whatever 'it' turns out to be, I have to multiply it by a million. It has to be affordable, it has to be scalable to 1 million and then, regarding the data types, we need to have at least a lot of different scientific communities saying, 'If you collect that, we will come.'"

Incorporating the genomics piece of the study is a bit more complicated than, for example, asking people to use a wearable device or submit urine and blood samples. It's not just the expense—Dishman says that although he has the funding to do it right now for the initial group of volunteers, there are more complex matters to consider.

For one thing, *All of Us* has promised to be transparent, meaning it will share information with its participants. When it comes to genetics, however, Dishman feels that this information is so sensitive, it needs to be delivered by someone who can explain what it means. "Quite frankly, there just aren't enough genetic counselors for us to tap into, to give responsible feedback to a million people yet," he says. "Sure, at the scale that I want to do this at, we need the cost of whole genome sequencing to come down, and I'm anticipating that will happen. More than that, though, it's the cost of responsibly giving the data back."

Dishman says they will be piloting both a whole genome sequencing study as well as a whole exome sequencing study (the exome consists of all the genome's exons, which are the coding portions of genes, the regions that get translated, or expressed, as proteins) in 2017. They will be inviting the participants along with genetic counselors, ethicists and other experts to help design some of the policies before making this available to large numbers of volunteers.

Come One, Come All

In contrast to typical medical research studies, *All of Us* is not focused on any particular disease: It's basically a "come as you are" study, inviting people of all ages and in all stages of health to participate. "We want a ton of people who aren't currently diagnosed with anything, or just have what they have," Dishman says. "Over a lifetime we're actually going to start to see what unfolds and which of these data types help you look back and say, 'Wow, we could have predicted that!' Or see correlations that we never knew. Here's how genetics plus environment plus upbringing sort of come together to lead toward disparities for this group, or a lack of resilience. Or why these other people under the same conditions thrive and do well."

Dishman says that the study will ultimately be the most diverse cohort ever assembled for any study, done by any nation. "We're aggressively recruiting people of all races, sexual preference and gender identities, those underrepresented in traditional biomedical research. We're looking for geographical diversity; we're recruiting in a mix of rural and urban areas and all points in between across the country," he explains. "Nobody else is doing it quite at the scale we are, but it's arguable that no other country could. America really is a melting pot, so we're able to get the diversity of genetics, race and ethnic and cultural backgrounds in one place."

When Dishman left Intel to pursue this study, he notes that many colleagues in the aging community accused him of "giving up" on them. But Dishman asserts nothing could be further from the truth. "First, we are going to be recruiting the old-old into our study. Second, I'm trying to understand aging not by just focusing on the aged, but on people of all ages, and what in the aging process ends up leading to disease or injury, or why do prevention strategies actually work for some or get held out for others? We're going to understand this at a scale that we've actually never been able to do before."

He quickly adds, however, that *All of Us* could provide valuable information on diseases like Alzheimer's, which directly impact the elder community. "For example, even though we're not recruiting people with Alzheimer's, some of them will have Alzheimer's when they start out or develop it later," Dishman says. "We will see the unfolding of the life experience with all of these telemetry data around their behavior and their clinical, socioeconomic and environmental conditions, and be able to go back and look and say, 'Hey, based on what outcomes happened, these were the big data combinatorial data types that actually could have taught us this or helped us understand that better. We'll know which ones were useful and what kind of correlations occurred between them."

Finding the Carrots and the Sticks

On the one hand, the more knowledge we obtain on lifestyle and disease, the better equipped we are to design preventive strategies and/or more effective treatments. On the other hand, all the knowledge in the world won't do any good if we can't get people to do their part. One of the goals of *All of Us* is to provide in-depth information on what behavior strategies work for specific populations. "The fact of the matter is, we really don't understand the science of persuasion and the science of motivation for the many varied differences of different kinds of people in the United States," Dishman notes. "It's not going to be one-size-fits-all, but there aren't an infinite number of strategies either. There are possibly 20 to 30 different strategies for different segments of the population that we need to know in order to personalize, localize and really understand the motivation to get them started on a prevention-based paradigm and a proactive-based paradigm. And then we need to know the mechanisms required to actually sustain that."

It will be decades before the *All of Us* project is completed and the vast quantities of data are analyzed. But Dishman predicts it will begin to spin off valuable information much earlier than that. "We can start to deliver interesting value to the scientific community in three or four years, even before we recruit the whole million, just from starting to have that much EHR data from so many diverse sources in one place," he says. "Then it just gets better and better after that, once we increase the number of people and add genomics."

Another way to think of this is the modern-day equivalent of the Framingham Heart Study, with a much larger sample size and much greater granularity of data. If you think of what the Framingham Study has taught us (we are continuing to harvest insights from it), imagine what we'll learn from this audacious trial.

One *Very* Brave Idea

In November 2015, the American Heart Association announced that Verily and AstraZeneca had joined them in seeking "one brave idea from a visionary leader" to "find a cure for coronary heart disease and improve cardiovascular health."

Heart disease is the #1 killer of both men and women in the United States and worldwide. Some 84 million people in the US have some form of heart disease: About 15 million of those have coronary heart disease (CHD), the buildup of plaque in the heart's arteries that can lead to heart attack, stroke and heart failure and that is the result of coronary artery disease (CAD). If we are ever to extend the healthspan, it is imperative that we deal with the heart disease epidemic. Because it is the most common form of heart disease, One Brave Idea focuses on CHD.

The AHA, Verily and AstraZeneca each contributed $25 million to the $75 million grant to fund five years of research, the largest single award ever given in the AHA's history. All three were looking for a new research model that would "provide a specialized team of interdisciplinary experts." The goal, as noted in the AHA press release, was to accelerate discovery "by removing the barriers and the silos that have plagued the traditional research model."

After nearly a year-long global search, the award went to a team headed by Calum MacRae, MD, PhD, chief of Cardiovascular Medicine at Brigham and Women's Hospital in Boston.

MacRae's career is the epitome of interdisciplinary: He is a cardiologist, geneticist and developmental biologist. Born in Scotland, MacRae came to Harvard Medical School in 1991 to work in the cardiovascular genetics lab of Jonathan and Christine Seidman. Later he moved to Mark Fishman's developmental biology lab at Massachusetts General Hospital. There, he pursued his study of human and zebrafish genetics (zebrafish are a species of fish that has genetics similar to humans).

In addition to being chief of cardiology at the Brigham and Women's Hospital, MacRae is a leading investigator at the Brigham and Women's Hospital Genomics Center, a principal faculty member at the Cardiovascular Center there and at the Harvard Stem Cell Institute, and an associate member at Broad Institute in Cambridge, Massachusetts. He is an inspiring individual to spend time with. We see the world alike and, at the time of this book's publication, are in the midst of detailed talks about an exciting collaboration.

MacRae's One Brave Idea team includes top researchers from MIT, Stanford University, Northeastern University and the University of Toronto, the principal investigator from the renowned Framingham Heart Study and two leaders of the Million Veteran Program. (The Million Veteran Program allows veterans in the VA Healthcare System to have their blood and health information used anonymously in medical research.) The team also includes a venture capitalist to devise new ways to get medical research funded, especially projects that may spin out from this one.

Their initial study will focus on people who have CHD in the family, putting them at higher risk for the disease. They will investigate what factors, if any, can predict early in life who will develop the disease and who will not. MacRae believes finding the answer will require a whole new approach to cardiac research, one that recognizes that human beings are much more than a heart pump and blood vessels. His team will be looking at the impact of phenotype on genetics, the "observable" characteristics of an individual that include everything from appearance to general health and behavior. (As of Spring 2017, they were laying the groundwork for the project and hope to move to clinical testing sometime in 2018.)

According to MacRae, "We need to develop new tools that deliberately target the areas of information content that we don't currently access. Instead of going deeper and deeper into the areas where we already have some information, which is the usual approach, we're deliberately picking areas where we know there's no information that's readily available."

Some of those targeted areas could include some seemingly "noncardiology" topics that MacRae believes could ultimately be significant. For example, he suggests that monitoring changes in an individual's body shape from childhood on could provide insight about that child's adult health. "The shape of your body is influenced by your development, by your growth, by how quickly you grow. And if we could understand better how people's shapes integrate all of the influences in early life, we would have a better index of what has happened to them by the time they get older," he says.

He adds, "You can make some inferences about what a person's calorie excess was just by measuring the person and knowing how long it took to develop that weight gain. On the other hand, if you understand it better in the context of other features, you may be able to discern what the underlying metabolic defect is that predisposed the person to a specific set of problems."

MacRae is also intrigued by the relationship between changes in facial characteristics and the onset of disease. There are some rare diseases in which changes in facial shape have been shown to be important but, so far, this has not been explored in terms of heart disease. "This is not based on any data, but it's perfectly surmisable that it might be relevant for a range of diseases. The way in which your face changes from when you're a baby to when you're an adult may actually tell us something about how your body's molecular pathways are set up," he says.

And he's already mulling over the kind of test that could capture this data. "You can do this very straightforwardly by taking a digital image and then extracting the information from that digital image if you have the right standardization," he says. "That's the type of holistic insight that we believe is important."

Most of all, MacRae wants to expand the way information is obtained about patients. He notes that with few exceptions most medicine is based on "static" information. For example, measurements of blood pressure, heart rate and assessments of overall health are typically done while the patient is sitting still on the examining table. It doesn't reveal much about "real-life" interactions.

To gain a real understanding of how the body reacts to particular situations, MacRae believes you need to "challenge" it, that is, track in real time the impact of something that elicits a response.

His lab has already developed a next-generation phenotyping platform for its ambulatory clinics, which, according to the lab's website, "is designed to test and validate new technologies bringing cell biology or physiology to the bedside."

These "experiments" could begin when the patient is sitting in the waiting room, using new tools that can gather important data even before the patient sees the doctor. "Why not have the ability to challenge a system that's important to you while you're sitting in the waiting room?" MacRae asks. "Why not challenge people's cognitive function? Why not challenge their mobility? Why not test their metabolic responses to some simple nutritional agent? Why not see how they respond to their medication—in real time?"

MacRae adds that the data could be automatically integrated into your medical record. "This way, your doctor would know much more about you as a biological entity and as a person after you'd spent some time in the waiting room—more than we know just by asking you questions." This approach will not only yield better information about patients, but it could help move the practice of medicine forward, which he feels is stuck in outmoded technology. For example, MacRae echoes a common complaint heard among patients: That doctors are so busy inputting data into their computers during a patient visit that they barely have time to observe or talk to the patient. "There's no other system on the planet where everybody has to type everything in," he asserts. "Even in a grocery store, the bar codes upload everything. Why don't we have a bar code in medicine, where we know what your basic biology looks like? It's frightening that we're so far behind every other field."

Breaking Down the Silos

Well before One Brave Idea, MacRae had been breaking down the silos that separated one medical specialty from another. Although he is not a dermatologist, he became fascinated by the fact that some cardiovascular disorders were closely associated with skin diseases. He veered off the traditional cardiology path by studying a disease characterized by skin problems on the palms and soles of the feet and—surprisingly—cardiac arrhythmias. He wondered whether there was more to cardiovascular disease than met the eye. MacRae reasoned that if cardiac researchers were only narrowly focused on the heart, what else were they missing? Could the pathway to heart disease actually begin on the skin . . . or somewhere else in the body? And would it be possible to get to the source of the disease early enough to sidestep the disease altogether?

He reached the conclusion that conventional cardiac medical research—like the practice of medicine itself—had become so overspecialized that it was often missing the big picture. In "Skin and Vascular Disease—Inside-Out/Outside-In," an article published online on May 31, 2017 in *JAMA Cardiology*, MacRae observes, "As medicine has evolved, incentives have created more specialized physicians who are consequently less capable of crossing the artificial boundaries that define their experience. Disease pathophysiology knows no such bounds."

Although specialists may be confined to their particular branch of science, MacRae notes, the human body doesn't work that way. "If you have inflammation in an artery, you may have inflammation in your skin, you may have inflammation in your joints, but nobody ever measures those things if you are being treated for arterial disease," he explains.

MacRae adds that because of this narrow focus, when a patient is examined by a specialist, "We measure very few things and we measure them often only in one system. But when you add them all up, there are really a very small number of endpoints and very poorly representative of what we know about biology today. These endpoints are almost all based on anatomy or physiology that was established 25, 50, even 100 years ago. We really haven't added very many new end points."

He attributes the knowledge gap to (1) the emphasis on genotype and genetics, which minimized phenotype, and (2) the rigid requirements of clinical trials. "In order to get clinical trials large enough to see an effect, you need to aggregate people who often have different variants of the same superficially similar disorder," he explains. In other words, the way medicine and research has been conducted in the past has made it difficult for people to maneuver beyond their specialties.

Part of his team's job, MacRae says, is figuring out what those new endpoints could be, and then designing tests to capture the right data. "I don't think the movement is necessarily reinventing the wheel, and it's also not rocket science. It's somewhere in between," he says. "It's basically saying, 'How can we systematically change the data collection that we have in medicine so that we actually are getting a comprehensive picture of the patient in quantifiable, computable terms that we can then use both to help with diagnosis, and therapy, but also to help with data entry?'"

MacRae says his research will take a multifactorial approach, looking at different phenomena normally ignored in conventional cardiology studies. Even before the One Brave Idea award, MacRae's lab had been developing new tools to better study the impact of phenotype on disease and health, which could be used in his study of families with CHD. These include looking more deeply at the skin-heart connection. Based on his earlier work, MacRae says that there are some very clear examples of things that can be measured on the skin that reflect the biology of the heart. "That's something that could be done noninvasively. It could be done in large numbers of people if we could build wearable devices that would allow that to happen."

Similarly, he adds, a closer look at the functionality of blood cells may also reveal problems earlier than conventional tests. For example, a defect in a pump that moves a particular ion in and out of blood cells could prove to be an early indicator of heart failure. "So why not measure that in the blood sample from cells in the peripheral blood to see if that reflects what's happening in the heart?" he asks. "In other words, can you characterize physiology and cell biology and molecular biology more broadly than just in the organs in which the disease has manifested, or the apparent disease has manifested? That's the type of thing that we're beginning to look at. All of the information that we collect is probably of some relevance to biology."

Going Upstream

Instead of relying on new and improved versions of tests that reveal what researchers already know about heart disease, MacRae's team will be developing some new tests of their own. His vision is to create a whole new way of identifying cardiovascular disease long before, as he puts it, "it comes to us," at the very first indication that something is going awry.

"We know what 'it' looks like when it comes to us, so let's go out looking for 'it' in the general population," MacRae says. For example, he notes that we routinely measure cholesterol, "But what we should be saying is, 'Let's try to understand what's upstream of cholesterol. And then, what's upstream of what's upstream of that?' And once we know that, we can then try and see what are the things that we can alter when you are only 3 or 5 years old that would change the way in which heart disease might develop."

MacRae notes that heart disease is ideal to study because there is a long lead-in to the predisease state, during which subtle changes are occurring in the body that could be indicative of trouble down the road. If we figure out what those changes may be early enough in life, it could make a big difference in future outcomes. MacRae says that having this knowledge could impact behavior. "We already have interventions that we know work, but work relatively poorly, and we know we could improve their efficacy just by applying them earlier," he explains. "Almost every behavioral intervention—in fact I don't think there's even one exception—has been shown to be more effective the earlier in life that you intervene. If you can just move the threshold so that you're detecting the disease earlier, then you're immediately improving the chances of changing behavior."

For example, MacRae says, "What if it was possible to detect a high risk of obesity in a very young child? What if you could actually say early in life, 'This person is going to end up with these complications.' You could potentially change behavior in ways that you can never change again after that child becomes a teenager."

He points out that, in some cases, if you don't get it early enough, the damage may already be done. "Some of those changes are not extrinsic; some of them may be intrinsic," MacRae explains. "It may be that your behavior is dictated because once you start to eat in a certain way, it patterns your body to eat again in similar ways. It may be that it changes the way that bacteria colonize your gut. You end up with bacteria that produce particular toxins that cause a disease that we don't really understand fully."

Understanding the Data

MacRae notes that in executing a study like this, there is a huge amount of potential data that can be collected, but not necessarily a huge amount of information. He admits that separating the nuggets of good information from the noise can be difficult, but not insurmountable. "If we can begin to collect data in an informed way, where we can challenge the system, understand the system at every level from single molecule all the way up to population, then that's *actually shedding insight into how all the big data fit together,"* he explains. But he also adds that the important organizing principle here is "the challenge."

"If you give a thousand people the same challenge and you get five different responses, that immediately lets me classify things in a much more robust way than just looking for patterns across cross-sectional evaluations over a long period of time," he says. "You're looking not only at the change, but you're looking at when it happened, how quickly it happened, how long it lasted, and you can begin to understand it at multiple levels. There's a cause and effect relationship, whereas just looking at static or cross-sectional information is much, much more difficult."

The One Brave Idea team will be gathering new kinds of data about health that could potentially require a whole new interpretation of heart disease. And that wouldn't surprise MacRae. "I think we're going to find that coronary heart disease is a relatively superficial characterization, that there are many different types of coronary disease. Who knows? Maybe we'll find that there are 10, 20, 30, 40, and that each of them has very discrete behaviors," he says. "This is one of the reasons why some people present with chronic chest pain or exertional angina and other people with seemingly the same underlying pathology drop dead as their first symptom. It's why some people get the disease when they're 20 and other people get it when they're 80. It's why in some people it involves one artery and in other people it involves a completely different artery with completely different consequences."

As far as I'm concerned, both Dishman and MacRae are true leaders, pushing the envelope in very important ways. There have been previous attempts to aggregate large cohorts of genetic information. While *All of Us* is bigger than any before, the real differentiator is the attempt to integrate quantitative physiologic data from wearables and the like. The most exciting aspect of One Brave Idea, in my opinion, is that Calum MacRae has surfaced the fact that our attempts to gather relevant data for clinical decision making are a full century behind our understanding of human biology. A perfect example is blood pressure taken with a traditional sphygmomanometer. He makes the case that this (and many other standard clinical data points) is outdated. Thinking like this is critical to our future of changing healthcare delivery for the better. As more data about human beings is collected, crunched, analyzed and incorporated into healthcare, connected health technologies will help close the gap between healthspan and lifespan.

Afterword

We're not getting any younger, either on an individual or societal level.

In the past century, we may have added more than a quarter-century to the lifespan, but we have not given much thought as to how to make the most of those additional 25 years of life. We must now dedicate ourselves to extending the healthspan to match the achievements in healthcare that we've made—and will continue to make—in extending the lifespan. It is critical that we turn our attention in this direction: If we continue to think of aging as a societal burden, we will bankrupt our economy and severely cripple our families and service infrastructure.

A two-part strategy is required—and we don't have a minute to lose.

First, we must start to look at aging as an opportunity rather than a burden. As we get older, we accumulate perspective, experience and wisdom. We must put structures in place to harness these attributes. A friend was in my office the other day talking about his innovative start-up and lamented to me: "There's a lot of ageism there. They've simply given up thinking that older people will use their services, saying 'old people don't get technology.'" As my colleague Jody Holtzman reminds us in Chapter 2, this is a market of more than 100 million people. If I was an investor in my friend's company, I would wonder whether my money was being put to good use when they ignore such a large market. Or, as my friend Charlotte Yeh puts it, if technologists love aging, they will design products and services that are welcomed by this demographic. However, if they love technology, they will most likely fail in this market. We have both an enormous economic opportunity and a design challenge.

We need more than a simple attitude adjustment. We need a whole society to adjust its attitude and to start looking at the over 65 population as an opportunity. Not only do older adults consume services, but if we create the right structures, they will add back to society in powerful, productive ways.

As I said in Chapter 7, the key to healthy longevity lies in three realms: *The first is maintaining a sense of purpose.* For many older adults, that sense of purpose will come in the form of contributions to the workforce for years—or even decades—beyond that arbitrary cutoff of age of 65. This self-reinforcing feedback loop will be a critical success factor. For others, it may be helping with family matters. In any case, matching the need for a sense of purpose with adding value back to society is a powerful concept. *The second key is social connections.* As was noted earlier in this book, and it bears repeating, isolation can be as detrimental to one's health as smoking 15 cigarettes a day. *The third is physical activity.* For some, this will be walking the dog, while for others it will be a two-hour trip to the gym each day. Of course, these three can be synergistic: Fulfilling your sense of purpose can result in both increased social connections and physical activity.

The second part of my two-part strategy has to do with the way we manage illness. As we age, we inevitably need more healthcare services. Part of this is purely related to chance—the longer you are alive, the more opportunity there is for something to go wrong—and another part is related to the natural slow deterioration of our physical being as time marches on. Thus, any plan to bring the healthspan into sync with the lifespan must include an intense focus on illness management.

Our healthcare system still functions best when dealing with acute conditions—automobile accidents, heart attacks, pneumonia and so on. Yet more than 70% of our costs are related to lifestyle. We need to revamp our system to be more focused on chronic illness management. This is not an option. No matter how much we promote purpose, social connections and physical activity, that growing cohort of folks over 65 will need care. We have already reached the point where we have more demand for healthcare services than we have providers and soon, as discussed throughout this book, we will reach the point where we don't even have enough young people to be caregivers for our elders. We have to create programs to keep people healthier longer. Making this happen is a complex task and includes changes that all stakeholders in healthcare delivery will need to make. Accordingly, we've covered this topic extensively throughout this book.

You may be surprised that I've yet to mention the role that technology will play. This is purposeful on my part. Technology is best applied in service to a problem and almost never does well when it leads, looking for a problem to solve. That said, technology can help achieve all of this. Going back to the three keys to longevity, technology has a central role to play in all three.

In terms of purpose, many technologically driven trends are coming to our aid at once. Increasingly, our work force is time- and place-independent. In February 2017, a *New York Times* piece reported on a Gallup poll that found, "More American employees are working remotely, and they are doing so for longer periods . . ." with 31 percent working remotely four to five days a week, up from 24 percent since 2012, according to the survey. The article concluded with another survey stat: that workers who spent 60 to 80 percent of their time away from the office had the highest rates of engagement. According to the poll: "In spite of the additional time away from managers and co-workers, they are the most likely of all employees to strongly agree that someone at work cares about them as a person, encourages their development and has talked to them about their progress." Sound familiar? We've had very similar feedback from patients participating in remote monitoring programs—feeling better connected to their provider, more engaged and in control of their health, and more satisfied with their care.

Likewise, technology now enables us to sell our knowledge by the slice. Both this and workers' independence are essential if we are to harness the work force potential of our aging society. While people rarely think of the "hard stop" retirement age as it was originally conceived when social security came into being, most people 65 and older inevitably want to do other things and most would prefer not to work full time. The time- and place-independent, technology-enabled gig economy is a perfect opportunity for us to add back much of that wisdom and experience I referred to earlier.

In terms of combating isolation, technologies like Skype and FaceTime (not to mention email and texting) enable us to routinely keep in touch with those who are geographically remote. These tools are a perfect antidote to isolation, as individuals become less able to physically move around.

Around 25% of older folks aged 55 and over own activity trackers. With the addition of engaging mobile apps, the future of physical activity as a public good looks very bright.

As it relates to chronic illness management, technology plays a central role. Healthcare providers can now video chat with their patients, securely message them, and monitor their vital signs in the home, all with technologies that are off-the-shelf and easily available. What has lagged are reimbursement models, provider attitudes and workflows. Yes, the technologies can get better too. Devices need to be easier to set up and the user design needs to be much better. Firms like Iora Health, profiled in Chapter 6, are leading the way in this new approach to providing care.

And we can't forget to address the use of technology for the inevitable time when we run out of people to care for our elderly. If we only think of one-to-one physical connections as the solution, this will happen sooner than we'd like to think. The technologies that will solve this are a combination of artificial intelligence (AI) and robotics.

Catching the healthspan up to the lifespan is a monumental task: It won't be easy. We have to make this a personal and societal priority. If we can turn aging into an opportunity, turn the system around so people give back as they grow older rather than become a burden, and turn our attention to more efficient management of chronic illness, we can make this happen.

Select Bibliography

Chapter 1: A New Kind of Old

"AARP, J.P. Morgan Asset Management Create First-of-its-Kind 'Innovation Fund' to Invest in Innovative Companies Focused on Improving the Lives of People 50-Plus." News release, AARP Press Room, October 1, 2015.

DeSilver, Drew. "More older Americans are working, and working more, than they used to." Pew Research Center, June 20, 2016.

"Facts for Features: Older Americans Month: May 2017. Newsroom, United States Census Bureau, April 10, 2017. https://www.census. gov/newsroom/facts-for-features/2017/cb17-ff08.html

Fogel, Alexander L., and Joseph C. Kvedar. "Simple Digital Technologies Can Reduce Health Care Costs." *Harvard Business Review*, November 14, 2016.

Healthy Aging Facts. National Council on Aging. https://www.ncoa. org/news/resources-for-reporters/get-the-facts/healthy-aging-facts/

Holt-Lunstad J, Smith TB, Baker M, et al. Loneliness and social isolation as risk factors for mortality: a meta-analytic review. *Perspect Psychol Sci.* 2015 Mar;10(2):227-37. doi: 10.1177/1745691614568352.

Japsen, Bruce. "Wearable Fitness Devices Attract More Than The Young and Healthy." *Forbes.com,* July 11, 2011.

Jenkins, JoAnn. *Disrupt Aging.* New York: Public Affairs, 2016.

Kvedar, Joseph C., Carol Colman, and Gina Cella. *The Internet of Healthy Things.* Boston: Partners Connected Health, 2015.

Kvedar JC, Fogel AL, Elenko E, Zohar D. Digital medicine's march on chronic disease. *Nat Biotechnol.* 2016 Mar;34(3):239-45.

Levine DM, Lipsitz SR, Linder JA. Trends in Seniors' Use of Digital Health Technology in the United States, 2011-2014. *JAMA.* 2016;316(5):538-540. doi:10.1001/jama.2016.9124.

"The Longevity Economy: How People Over 50 Are Driving Economic and Social Value in the US." A report prepared by Oxford Economics for AARP. September 2016.

Moore, Geoffrey A. *Crossing the Chasm: Marketing and Selling High-Tech Products to Mainstream Customers.* New York: HarperCollins, 1991.

Smith, Aaron. "Older Adults and Technology Use." Pew Research Center, April 3, 2014.

Steverman, Ben. "'I'll Never Retire.' Americans Break Record for Working Past 65." *Bloomberg News,* May 13, 2016.

Chapter 2: The Challenge—and Opportunity—of an Aging World

"2017 Alzheimer's Disease Facts and Figures." Alzheimer's Association. www.alz.org/facts/

"Ageing and Health." World Health Organization. Fact Sheet No. 404, September 2015. http://www.who.int/mediacentre/factsheets/fs404/en/

Choi SH, Kim YH, Quinti L, Tanzi RE, et al. 3D culture models of Alzheimer's disease: a road map to a "cure-in-a-dish". *Mol Neurodegener.* 2016 Dec 9;11(1):75. doi: 10.1186/s13024-016-0139-7.

Cubanski, Juliette, and Tricia Neuman. "The Facts on Medicare Spending and Financing." The Henry J. Kaiser Family Foundation, July 18, 2017.

"Dementia: a public health priority." World Health Organization and Alzheimer's Disease International, 2012. http://www.who.int/mental_health/publications/dementia_report_2012/en/

Diabetes: At a Glance Fact Sheets. Centers for Disease Control and Prevention, July 25, 2016. https://www.cdc.gov/chronicdisease/resources/publications/aag/diabetes.htm

Ding D, Lawson KD, Kolbe-Alexander TL, et al. The economic burden of physical inactivity: a global analysis of major non-communicable diseases." *Lancet.* 2016 Sep 24;388(10051):1311-24.

Global Burden of Disease Health Financing Collaborator Network. Evolution and patterns of global health financing 1995–2014: development assistance for health, and government, prepaid private, and out-of-pocket health spending in 184 countries. *Lancet.* 2017 May 20;389(10083):1981-2004.

Greeley, Michael. "Life Expectancy Gradient . . . Role of Healthcare Technology." *On the Flying Bridge,* November 2, 2016.

Hafner, Katie. "As Population Ages, Where Are the Geriatricians?" *New York Times*, January 25, 2016.

He, Wan, Daniel Goodkind, and Paul Kowal. "An Aging World: 2015." International Population Reports. United States Census Bureau, March 2016. https://www.census.gov/content/dam/Census/library/publications/2016/demo/p95-16-1.pdf.

Minter MR, Zhang C, Leone V, et al. Antibiotic-induced perturbations in gut microbial diversity influences neuro-inflammation and amyloidosis in a murine model of Alzheimer's disease. *Sci Rep.* 2016 Jul 21;6: 30028. doi: 10.1038/srep30028.

"New Research Confirms Looming Physician Shortage." News release, Association of American Medical Colleges, April 5, 2016.

"Older Persons' Health." Centers for Disease Control and Prevention, January 19, 2917. https://www.cdc.gov/nchs/fastats/older-american-health.htm

Taylor, Adam. "It's official: Japan's population is dramatically shrinking." *Washington Post*, February 26, 2016.

Wagner SL, Rynearson KD, Duddy SK, et al. Pharmacological and Toxicological Properties of the Potent Oral γ-Secretase Modulator

BPN-15606. *J Pharmacol Exp Ther.* 2017 Jul; 362(1):31-44. doi: 10.1124/jpet.117.240861.

"World Alzheimer Report 2015:The Global Impact of Dementia." Alzheimer's Disease International, London, August 2015.

Chapter 3: The Chicken or the Egg

"Healthcare's Digital Divide Widens, Black Book Consumer Survey." News release, *Newswire.com*, January 3, 2017.

Ipsos Global Trends Survey on Connected Health 2017. "Connected Health Device Recommended by Doctor."

Ipsos Global Trends Survey on Connected Health 2015. "Connected Health Device Recommended by Insurance Company."

Lally, Dennis. "Why Tech Firms Can't Afford to Ignore Seniors." *Fortune.com,* September 6, 2016.

"Survey Finds Physicians Enthusiastic About Digital Health Innovation." American Medical Association, September 26, 2016.

Chapter 4: From Reactive to Proactive: Taking the First Steps

Akinbosoye, Osayi, Darius Taylor, Jenny Jiang, et al. "The Relationship Between Digital Health Program Activity Tracking and Medication Adherence Among Members Age 50+ Years." Presented at the Academy of Managed Care Pharmacy Annual Meeting, April 19-22, 2016, San Francisco, CA.

Akinbosoye, Osayi, Jenny Jiang, Michael Taitel, et al, "The Association between Use of a Community Pharmacy's Mobile Pill Reminder App and Medication Adherence." Presented at the Society of Behavioral Medicine 37th Annual Meeting, March 30-April 2, 2016, Washington, DC.

Brody, Jane E. "The Cost of Not Taking Your Medicine." *New York Times*, April 17, 2017.

Jethwani, Kamal, Julie Kvedar, and Joseph Kvedar. "Behavioral Phenotyping: A Tool for Personalized Medicine." *Personalized Medicine.* 2010;7(6): 689-693.

"Three-year Study Shows Engagement in Wellness Program Lowers Health Claims Costs, Improves Work Productivity." News release, *Business Wire*, March 29, 2016.

Chapter 5: Reading People

Khatchadourian, Raffi. "We Know How You Feel." *The New Yorker*, January 19, 2015.

Maor, Elad, Jaskanwal D. Sara, Lilach O. Lerman, et al. The Sound of Atherosclerosis: Voice Signal Characteristics are Independently Associated with Coronary Artery Disease. *Circulation.* Nov 11, 2016;134, Issue Suppl 1:A15840.

Miner A, Milstein A, Schueller S, et al. Smartphone-Based Conversational Agents and Responses to Questions About Mental Health, Interpersonal Violence, and Physical Health. *JAMA Intern Med.* 2016;176(5):619-25. doi:10.1001/jamainternmed.2016.0400.

Chapter 6: Managing Chronic Disease

Castro Sweet CM, Vinay Chiguluri, Rajiv Gumpina, et al. Outcomes of a Digital Health Program With Human Coaching for Diabetes Risk Reduction in a Medicare Population. *Journal of Aging and Health.* Article first published online: January 24, 2017.

Chen F, Su W, Becker SH, et al. Clinical and Economic Impact of a Digital, Remotely-Delivered Intensive Behavioral Counseling Program on Medicare Beneficiaries at Risk for Diabetes and Cardiovascular Disease. *PLOS One.* 2016 Oct 5;11(10)e0163627. doi:10.1371/journal pone 0163627. eCollction 2016.

Chi N, Demiris G, Thompson H, Lazar A, et al. The Usability of a Digital Companion Pet for Older Adults with Mild Cognitive Impairment. *Gerontologist.* 2016.56 (Suppl_3):566.

Chi N, Sparks O, Lin S, et al. Pilot testing a digital pet avatar for older adults. *Geriatr Nurs.* 2017 May 4. pii: S0197-4572(17)30106-4. doi: 10.1016/j.gerinurse.2017.04.002. [Epub ahead of print].

Demiris G, Thompson HJ, Lazar A, et al. Evaluation of a Digital Companion for Older Adults with Mild Cognitive Impairment. *JAMA Annu Symp Proc.* 2017 Feb 10;2016:496-503. eCollection 2016.

"Fitbit Announces Adam Pellegrini as Vice President of Digital Health." News release, *Business Wire*, August 1, 2016.

Gawande, Atul. "The Hot Spotters: Can We Lower Medical Costs by Giving the Neediest Patients Better Care?" *The New Yorker*, January 24, 2011.

Gregg EW, Sattar N, Ali MK. The changing face of diabetes complications. *Lancet Diabetes Endocrinol.* 2016 Jun;4(6):537-47. doi: 10.1016/S2213-8587(16)30010-9. Epub 2016 May 4.

Marcantonio ER. Postoperative delirium: a 76-year-old woman with delirium following surgery." *JAMA.* 2012 Jul 4;308(1):73-81. doi:10.1001/jama.2012.6857.

McCusker J, Cole MG, Dendukuri N, et al. Does delirium increase hospital stay? *J Am Geriatr Soc.* 2003 Nov;51(11):1539-46.

"Preventing Falls in Hospitals." US Department of Health & Human Services, 2017. Publication: 13-0015-EF.

"The Staggering Costs of Diabetes." American Diabetes Association. http://www.diabetes.org/diabetes-basics/statistics/infographics/adv-staggering-cost-of-diabetes.html

"Statistics About Diabetes." July 19, 2017. American Diabetes Association. http://www.diabetes.org/diabetes-basics/statistics/

Wexler, Sharon, Lin Drury, and Marie-Claire Roberts. "The Use of an Avatar Virtual Service Animal to Improve Hospital Outcomes in Older Adults." Abstract presented at the Gerontological Society of America's 69th Annual Scientific Meeting in New Orleans, LA, November 2016.

Wexler SS, Drury L, Pollack C. "The Use of an Avatar Virtual Service Animal to Improve Outcomes in Hospitalized Older Adults." Presented at NICHE Annual Conference, Austin, TX, April, 2017.

Chapter 7: Putting the "Well" Back into Well-being

Case, Ann, and Angus Deaton. "Mortality and morbidity in the 21st Century." Prepared for the Brookings Panel on Economic Activity, March 23-24, 2017.

Chihuri S, Melenz TJ, DiMaggio CJ, et al. Driving Cessation and Health Outcomes in Older Adults. *Jour Am Geriatr Soc.* 2016 Feb;64(2):332-41. doi: 10.1111/jgs.13931. Epub 2016 Jan 19.

Hobbs WR, Burke M, Christakis NA, et al. Online social integration is associated with reduced mortality risk." *Proc Natl Acad Sci U.S.A.* 2016 Nov 15;113(46):12980-12984.

Kim ES, Hagan KA, Goodstein F, et al. Optimism and Cause-Specific Morality: A Prospective Cohort Study. *Am J Epidemiol.* 2017 Jan 1;185(1):21-29. doi: 10.1093/aje/kww182. Epub 2016 Dec 7.

Kim ES, Konrath S. Volunteering is prospectively associated with health care use among older adults. *Soc Sci Med.* 2016 Jan;149:122-9. doi: 10.1016/j.socscimed.2015.11.043. Epub 2015 Nov 30.

Kim ES, Kubzansky LD, Soo J, et al. Maintaining Healthy Behavior: a Prospective Study of Psychological Well-Being and Physical Activity. *Ann Behav Med.* 2017 Jun;51(3):337-347. doi: 10.1007/s12160-016-9856-y.

Kim ES, Strecher VJ, Ryff CD. Purpose in life and use of preventive health care services. *Proc Natl Acad Sci U.S.A.* 2014 Nov 18;111(46):16331-6. doi: 10.1073/pnas.1414826111. Epub 2014 Nov 3.

Larson, Jeremy D. "Letter of Recommendation: Hasbro Joy for All." *New York Times*, March 24, 2016.

Levy, Becca. Stereotype Embodiment: A Psychosocial Approach to Aging. *Curr Dir Psychol Sci.* 2009 Dec 1;18(6):332–336.

Levy BR, Ferrucci L, Zonderman AB, et al A culture-brain link: Negative age stereotypes predict Alzheimer's disease biomarkers. *Psychol Aging.* 2016 Feb;31(1):82-8. doi: 10.1037/pag0000062. Epub 2015 Dec 7.

Levy BR, Leifheit-Limson E. The stereotype-matching effect: greater influence on functioning when age stereotypes correspond to outcomes. *Psychol Aging.* 2009 Mar;24(1):230-33. doi: 10.1037/a0014563.

Levy BR, Slade MD, Kunkel SR, et al. Longevity increased by positive self-perceptions of aging. *J Pers Soc Psychol.* 2002 Aug;83(2):261-70.

Lilleston, Randy. "The Major Health Issue Affecting Seniors: Isolation and Loneliness Have Serious Consequences." AARP, May 18, 2017.

Lin, Frank R., and Marilyn Albert. Hearing Loss and Dementia—Who's Listening? *Aging Ment Health.* 2014 Aug;18(6):671-673. doi: 10.1080/13607863.2014.915924.

Peterson, Janey C., Mary E. Charlson, Zachary Hoffman, et al. Randomized Controlled Trial of Positive Affect Induction to Promote Physical Activity After Percutaneous Coronary Intervention. *Arch Intern Med.* 2012 Feb 27;172(4) 329-336. Published online 2012 Jan 23. doi: 10.1001/archinternmed.2011.1311.

Steptoe, Andrew, Angus Deaton, and Arthur A. Stone. "Subjective wellbeing, health and ageing." *Lancet.* 2015 Feb 14;385(9968):640-648. Published online 2014 Nov 6. doi: 10.1016/S014-67036(13)61489-0.

Sun JS, Kim ES, Smith J. Positive Self-Perceptions of Aging and Lower Rate of Overnight Hospitalization in the US Population Over Age 50. *Psychosom Med.* 2017 Jan;79(1):81-90. doi: 10.1097/PSY.0000000000000364.

Valtorta NK, Kanaan M, Gilbody S, et al. Loneliness and social isolation as risk factors for coronary heart disease and stroke: systematic review and meta-analysis of longitudinal observational studies. *Heart.* 2016 Jul 1;102(13):1009-16. Epub 2016 Apr 18.

Chapter 8: The Art and Science of Caregiving

"Caregiver Health: A Population at Risk." Family Caregiver Alliance. https://www.caregiver.org/caregiver-health

"Caregivers & Technology: What They Want and Need." AARP Project Catalyst, April 11, 2016. http://www.aarp.org/content/dam/aarp/home-and-family/personal-technology/2016/04/Caregivers-and-Technology-AARP.pdf.

"Caregiving Innovation Frontiers." AARP, January 2016. http://www.aarp.org/content/dam/aarp/home-and-family/personal-technology/2016-01/2016-Caregiving-Innovation-Frontiers-Infographics-AARP.pdf.

Leiber, Nick. "Europe Bets on Robots to Help Care for Seniors." *Bloomberg Businessweek*, March 17, 2016.

Mims, Christopher. "Your Next Friend Could Be a Robot." *Wall Street Journal,* October 9, 2016.

Sundar, S. Shyam, Eun Hwa Jung, T. Franklin Waddell, et al. "Cheery companions or serious assistants? Role and demeanor congruity as predictors of robot attraction and use intentions among senior citizens." *International Journal of Human-Computer Studies*, Volume *97*, January 2017, Pages 88-97.

Chapter 9: Cracking the Code for Healthy Longevity

"Beta Testing Begins for NIHs *All of Us* Research Program." National Institutes of Health, June 5, 2017.

"Calum MacRae Receives $75 Million to Pursue 'One Brave Idea' to Beat Coronary Heart Disease." *American Heart Association News*, October 5, 2016.

MacRae, CA. Skin and Vascular Disease—Inside-Out/Outside In." *JAMA Cardiol*. 2017 May 31. doi: 10.1001/jamacardio.2017.1420. [Epub ahead of print].

Eisenstadt, Leah. "What is exome sequencing?" Broadminded Blog. The Broad Institute, October 15, 2010. https://www.broadinstitute.org/blog/what-exome-sequencing

"One Brave Idea: Seeking a Cure for Coronary Heart Disease and Its Devastating Consequences." AHA/ASA Newsroom, Dallas, TX, January 14, 2016.

"Selection of Eric Dishman as Director of the Precision Medicine Initiative Cohort Program." National Institutes of Health, April 10, 2016.

Afterword

"Building a Better Tracker: Older Consumers Weigh In on Activity and Sleep Monitoring Devices." AARP Project Catalyst. http://www.aarp.org/content/dam/aarp/home-and-family/personal-technology/2015-07/innovation-50-project-catalyst-tracker-study-AARP.pdf.

Chokshi, Niraj. "Out of the Office: More People Are Working Remotely, Survey Finds." *New York Times*, February 15, 2017.

Index

Empactica, 8

employers, pay-for-performance insurance models and, 66

employment
among Japanese elderly, 31–32
as source of purpose, 161

engagement. *See* social connectedness

environment, genetics *vs.*, 25

ePAL, 97

EQ (emotional quotient), 112

exercise
Alzheimer's and, 46
connected health and, 53
Fitbit, 147–152
Iora Health's approach to planning/monitoring, 135
longevity and, 228
walking, 46, 47, 65–66, 204–205
well-being and, 164–165

exome sequencing study, 213

expenditures. *See* healthcare costs

Exponential Medicine, 37

Facebook, 6, 155, 176

FaceTime, 10, 230

Facial Action Coding System (FACS), 115

facial characteristics, CHD and, 219

facial expressions, as source of medical data, 112–116

falling, 18, 145, 146, 157–158, 168, 187

Family Caregiving Institute, 186–189

FDA (Food and Drug Administration), 59, 62–63

Feast, Joshua, 106–107

fee-for-service, 26

Fernandopulle, Rushika, 124, 127, 134–139

Ferris, Timothy G., 134

Fischer, Ted, 153, 170–174

Fishman, Mark, 217

F.I.T. walking goals, 65–66

Fitbit, 147–152

Fitbit Charge2, 150

Fitbit Health Solutions, 149

Flare Capital, 191

Flare Capital Partners, 32, 33, 135

Food and Drug Administration (FDA), 59, 62–63

Fowler, James, 155

Frankl, Viktor, 161–162

Friedman, Eric, 147

Frydman, Gilles, 176

future issues

About the Authors

Joseph C. Kvedar, MD

Joe Kvedar, vice president of Connected Health at Partners HealthCare in Boston, is creating a new model of healthcare delivery, developing innovative strategies to move care from the hospital or doctor's office into the day-to-day lives of patients. He is internationally recognized as a pioneer and visionary in the field of connected health.

Carol Colman

Carol Colman is the co-author of more than two dozen books on health, wellness, antiaging and technology, including numerous *New York Times* and national bestsellers. She lives in Brooklyn, New York.

Gina Cella

Gina Cella is the principal of Boston-based Cella Communications, a public relations firm representing leaders in the field of healthcare, promoting cutting-edge personal health technologies, provider organizations and biotech/pharma companies for the past two decades.

Made in the USA
Middletown, DE
13 November 2020

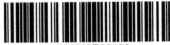